# The Ritalin-Free Child

## Managing Hyperactivity &
## Attention Deficits
## Without Drugs

### by Diana Hunter

Consumer Press
Fort Lauderdale, Florida

*For Tony and Brenden*

Published by:
**Consumer Press**
13326 Southwest 28th Street, Suite 102
Fort Lauderdale, FL 33330-1102 U.S.A.

**Library of Congress Cataloging in Publication Data**
Hunter, Diana, 1961-
The ritalin-free child: managing hyperactivity and attention deficits without drugs/by Diana Hunter. — 1st ed.
    p.    cm.
Includes index.
1. Attention-deficit hyperactivity disorder—Alternative treatment.
I. Title.
RJ506.H9H86    1995                                    95-47004
618.92'858906—dc20                                        CIP

ISBN 0-9628336-8-1        $12.95  Softcover

10  9  8  7  6  5
Printed in the United States of America

# The Ritalin-Free Child

# Contents

# Acknowledgements

Appreciation is gratefully extended to Laura Sotera, Garry Spear, Diane Lentini, Susie Gonzalez, Sandra Sobel, Joseph Pappas, Nancy Andrews, Jackie Gran, Kate Warner, Cindy Bradley, Armando Gonzalez, and Debbie Brechner for their efforts and expertise.

Special thanks to the many parents, children, and professionals who willingly provided suggestions, answers, and insight to make this book a reality, as well as to the American Psychiatric Association for granting permission of reprint.

*The use of male pronouns throughout this book does not reflect chauvinism. The decision for this usage was based on the fact that, according to research, more males than females are affected by hyperactivity and inattention.*

# Introduction

Millions of American children are affected by problems related to hyperactivity and inattention. Some face only a few minor difficulties, while others experience numerous cognitive and social struggles both at home and at school. Many have excessive energy and suffer from lack of concentration, distractibility, impulsivity, anxiousness, and exaggerated emotions.

There is considerable controversy as to whether the symptoms these children experience are actually attributable to a disorder. Although no medical cause has been verified, a number of behavioral scientists and medical professionals believe that such behaviors are caused by an abnormality in brain function. Skeptics, on the other hand, contest that the brain function of children with these symptoms may be "different," rather than "abnormal." Nevertheless, Attention Deficit Hyperactivity Disorder (ADHD) has become the most commonly known "psychiatric disorder" affecting children, and continues to be diagnosed with increasing frequency.

Regardless of the cause, many children whose difficulties stem from hyperactivity and inattention can benefit from some form of intervention. While a number of experts agree that a combination of medication, group and family therapy, psychotherapy, behavioral modification, and appropriate educational guidance can improve the symptoms common to hyperactivity and attention deficits, few exact a continual treatment program free of drug therapy. Yet a need exists.

There are a number of reasons why drug therapy may not be suitable as either a temporary or long-term course of action for hyperactivity and inattention. Among the most common is a child's sensitivity to one or more of the medications routinely prescribed for these conditions. Drug interactions with medication for asthma, epilepsy, high blood pressure, Tourette's syndrome, or other disorders are also causes for avoidance. For some children, medication prescribed for hyperactivity and inattention proves to be ineffective, or later becomes ineffective. Others don't have symptoms severe enough to need medication. And finally, there are the many parents who do not want their children to receive drug therapy.

Although medication may be helpful or even necessary for improvement in some cases, drug-free management often proves to be both effective and beneficial. The main factor in the success of a drug-free plan is selecting one which is most appropriate for the child. Other essential factors include parental awareness, understanding, patience, ongoing communication, positive attitude, and consistency.

With effort, children who are overly active and lack focus can be taught to use their energy in positive, productive ways. Exercising a child's mental muscle, while teaching the child to exercise it himself, is the key. In this way, parents and teachers can develop a success plan for hyperactive and inattentive children, rather than a drug regimen.

This book was written to give a different perspective on managing hyperactivity and inattention. Its purpose is to provide insight into the many ways these behaviors can be managed without drug therapy. Its strategy is to show parents and teachers how to teach children effective ways to turn their difficulties into assets. Its goal is to help hyperactive and inattentive children find the lasting confidence and self-esteem they need in order to lead happy, fulfilling, and productive lives.

Diana Hunter

# Chapter One

## *Attention Deficit Hyperactivity Disorder*
### An In-Depth Look At The Diagnosis Of The Decade

Attention Deficit Hyperactivity Disorder, commonly known as ADHD, is one of the most controversial and misunderstood conditions of our time. While many people believe ADHD to be a brain-based disease affecting between 2 and 3 million American children, others see it as a ploy to diagnose countless youths with a condition that doesn't really exist.

A number of skeptics insist that the symptoms of ADHD are within the limits of "normal" human behavior. Some suggest that ADHD is not a disease or disorder at all, but rather inherited traits of metabolism and personality carried down from previous generations. Even major research in which variations in glucose metabolism have been indicated as a possible cause of ADHD symptoms has come under fire. Skeptics contend that if one person's brain uses more glucose than another's, it may simply be a difference and not a deficit. In each of these cases, arguments against the use of drug therapy exist.

Amidst the controversy, research on ADHD continues. Scientists and medical researchers hope to one day provide concrete evidence as to what causes hyperactivity and related behaviors. In the meantime, parents can effectively help their hyperactive and inattentive children by teaching them how to use their energies in productive, focused ways.

The remainder of this chapter provides insight into how ADHD evolved, as well as a look at the behaviors commonly seen in affected children. Additionally, it recognizes why symptoms alone are not enough to confirm a diagnosis.

## History & Background

Although ADHD is now diagnosed with some frequency—enough to attract being labeled "The Diagnosis of the Decade"—it is not at all new. As far back as the mid-1800s children were described as having many of the same behaviors that characterize ADHD today.

Up until approximately 1960, ADHD-type symptoms were believed to be directly related to various forms of brain damage. Brain infections (encephalitis), measles, lead poisoning, and brain injuries—including those believed to occur during pregnancy or birth—were cited as the most likely causes. During this time the terms "hyperkinetic impulse disorder" and "minimal brain damage" were used to describe the behavioral and cognitive difficulties of hyperactive and inattentive children.

The 1960s brought about the realization that the brain damage theory was lacking in several areas. New research stemmed as a result, and investigation began into other possibilities. Hyperactivity, learning disabilities, and dyslexia were among those recognized as probable causes.

The 1970s yielded a downpour of investigation into hyperactivity from many major researchers. Thousands of related research studies were performed and published. During this decade, attention deficits were first recognized as a plausible cause of difficulty among children both with and without hyperactivity.

By the 1980s the development of precise diagnostic criteria became the focus. This most active period presented more research and controversy than any prior decade. During this time the term Attention Deficit Disorder (ADD) came into existence. It was replaced by Attention Deficit Hyperactivity Disorder toward the end of the decade.

Today, research on hyperactivity, inattention, and related behaviors continues. Further changes in criteria and description are likely as studies and surveys reveal new findings and statistics. Below is an overview of some of the developments that led to ADHD as it is presently known:

1845    German physician Heinrich Hoffmann wrote comical children's stories designed to teach moral lessons. He depicted characteristics of ADHD in his characters, whose actions were inspired by actual children.

1902    At the turn of the century British pediatri-
        cian George F. Still reported ADHD-like
        symptoms in children he was treating in his
        practice. Dr. Still believed these symptoms
        to have a biological basis.

1923    Researcher F.G. Ebaugh maintained that
        symptoms common to ADHD required not
        only acknowledgement, but also ongoing
        intervention and appropriate treatment
        from more than one area of medicine. His
        recommendations were based on studies of
        children who became brain-damaged after
        contracting encephalitis, a viral infection of
        the nervous system which causes inflamma-
        tion of the brain. Later reports showed
        significant improvement in a number of
        postencephalitic children after uncomplicat-
        ed behavioral programs were implemented.

1937    Research done by Dr. Charles Bradley
        indicated that hyperactivity might have a
        neurological basis. This conclusion was
        reached after Bradley reported behavioral
        changes in half of the hyperactive children
        he was treating with stimulant medication.

1943    Studies on soldiers who exhibited behavioral
        changes after sustaining brain injuries led
        researchers to further their investigations on

brain damage as a possible cause of behavior-related problems.

**1960**    The possibility of hyperactivity as a biologically-based neurological disorder was explored by Stella Chess and other researchers. Chess in particular believed the symptoms of hyperactivity to be physiologically oriented, rather than caused by brain damage or poor parenting.

**1966**    Many school-age children began being diagnosed as having *minimal brain dysfunction*. This distressing description, designated by a U.S. Department of Health, Education and Welfare task force, lasted only two short years.

**1968**    The American Psychiatric Association rendered its views by including *hyperkinetic disorder of childhood* in the association's second edition of the Diagnostic and Statistical Manual of Mental Disorders, or DSM-II.

**1972**    Researcher Virginia Douglas and others cited hyperactivity combined with inattention and impulsivity—rather than hyperactivity alone—as the cause of behavioral and cognitive difficulties for many children.

1980    A new version of the American Psychiatric
        Association's Diagnostic and Statistical
        Manual of Mental Disorders (DSM-III) was
        published, this time describing two forms of
        the condition: Attention Deficit Disorder
        (ADD) and Attention Deficit Disorder with
        Hyperactivity (ADD-H). Many people credit
        noted researcher Virginia Douglas with influ-
        encing this change of name.

1987    A revised version of DSM-III (DSM-III-R)
        was released, listing the name as it is known
        today—Attention Deficit Hyperactivity
        Disorder (ADHD). Another category, Un-
        differentiated Attention Deficit Disorder
        (UADD), was added to include children
        with attention deficits and related difficul-
        ties who were not hyperactive.

1994    The latest version of the American Psychi-
        atric Association's Diagnostic and Statistical
        Manual of Mental Disorders (DSM-IV) was
        published. This edition maintains the name
        Attention Deficit Hyperactivity Disorder,
        although it provides a more vivid descrip-
        tion of symptoms with specific subtypes.

Over the years, ADHD has sustained many other
names in addition to those already mentioned. Among
them are hyperactivity, hyperactive child syndrome,

brain damage syndrome, minimal cerebral dysfunction, minor cerebral dysfunction, postencephalitic disorder, hyperkinesis, dyslexia, and learning disabilities. This lengthy list has added to the skepticism and uncertainty that surrounds ADHD, and emphasizes the need for a definitive cause obtained from valid research.

Throughout this book, the acronym ADHD is used as a general description of the difficulties children may encounter due to hyperactivity and inattentiveness.

## Recognizing ADHD

Another hurdle in proving the validity of ADHD as a true "disorder" is its lack of exact, consistent characteristics. Each affected child can exhibit different symptoms, in varying degrees. Additionally, while the core symptoms of ADHD are inattention, impulsivity, and hyperactivity, a properly diagnosed child need not display all three.

DSM-IV lists various diagnostic criteria for each subtype of ADHD in its guidelines. It is noted that several symptoms must consistently appear for more than six months in order for a diagnosis to be considered. Additionally, these behavioral symptoms must have been present to some extent before age seven, and cannot be attributed to a specific cause, such as extreme stress, depression, or a reaction to medication. The diagnostic criteria for ADHD as listed in DSM-IV are included in the following pages.

# Diagnostic Criteria For Attention Deficit Hyperactivity Disorder

A. Either (1) or (2):

(1) six (or more) of the following symptoms of inattention have persisted for at least 6 months to a degree that is maladaptive and inconsistent with developmental level:

*Inattention*

(a) often fails to give close attention to details or makes careless mistakes in schoolwork, work, or other activities

(b) often has difficulty sustaining attention in tasks or play activities

(c) often does not seem to listen when spoken to directly

(d) often does not follow through on instructions and fails to finish schoolwork, chores, or duties in the workplace (not due to oppositional behavior or failure to understand instructions)

(e) often has difficulty organizing tasks and activities

(f) often avoids, dislikes, or is reluctant to engage in tasks that require sustained mental effort (such as schoolwork or homework)

(g) often loses things necessary for tasks or activities (e.g., toys, school assignments, pencils, books, or tools)

(h) is often easily distracted by extraneous stimuli

(i) is often forgetful in daily activities

(2) six (or more) of the following symptoms of hyperactivity-impulsivity have persisted for at least 6 months to a degree that is maladaptive and inconsistent with developmental level:

*Hyperactivity*

(a) often fidgets with hands or feet or squirms in seat

(b) often leaves seat in classroom or in other situations in which remaining seated is expected

(c) often runs about or climbs excessively in situations in which it is inappropriate (in adolescents or adults, may be limited to subjective feelings of restlessness)

(d) often has difficulty playing or engaging in leisure activities quietly

(e) is often "on the go" or often acts as if "driven by a motor"

(f) often talks excessively

*Impulsivity*
>    (g) often blurts out answers before questions have been completed
>    (h) often has difficulty awaiting turn
>    (i) often interrupts or intrudes on others (e.g., butts into conversations or games)

B. Some hyperactive-impulsive or inattentive symptoms that caused impairment were present before age 7 years.

C. Some impairment from the symptoms is present in two or more settings (e.g., at school (or work) and at home).

D. There must be clear evidence of clinically significant impairment in social, academic, or occupational functioning.

E. The symptoms do not occur exclusively during the course of a Pervasive Developmental Disorder, Schizophrenia, or other Psychotic Disorder and are not better accounted for by another mental disorder (e.g. Mood Disorder, Anxiety Disorder, Dissociative Disorder, or a Personality Disorder).

Code based on type:
>    314.01 **Attention-Deficit/Hyperactivity Disorder, Combined Type:**
>    If both Criteria A1 and A2 are met for the past 6 months
>    314.00 **Attention-Deficit/Hyperactivity Disorder, Predominantly Inattentive Type:**
>    If Criterion A1 is met but Criterion A2 is not met for the past 6 months
>    314.01 **Attention-Deficit/Hyperactivity Disorder, Predominantly Hyperactive-Impulsive Type:**
>    If Criterion A2 is met but Criterion A1 is not met for the past 6 months

Coding note: For individuals (especially adolescents and adults) who currently have symptoms that no longer meet full criteria, "In Partial Remission" should be specified.

The purpose of these criteria is to help provide some direction in assessing whether a child has ADHD.

These guidelines are general, and are by no means the last word in making a diagnosis. In fact, many people debate whether these criteria are accurate.

When considering each characteristic, it is important to remember that the behaviors must occur more frequently than in most children of the same age. The behaviors should also be age-appropriate, meaning that they need to fit the level of capability which is common to that age. One should also keep developmental and experience-based differences in mind.

Children with ADHD may also demonstrate other behaviors. Those that follow are often reported by parents, teachers, and others who provide assistance and intervention.

### Exaggerated Emotional States

Extreme happy and sad moods are common among ADHD children. They may have drastic mood swings, known in medical arenas as "emotional lability," being irritable one moment and delighted the next.

### Maladaptation

New schedules and situations that require change can cause difficulty for the ADHD child. Those with severe attention deficits generally have the most trouble in this area.

### Hypersensitivity

ADHD children are often sensitive to noise, light, and smells. Buzzing, whistling, or other sounds may easily irritate them (unless they are the source). The scent of certain foods and perfumes can be particularly annoying. Smells most people hardly notice can be very vivid to an ADHD child.

### Noncompliance & Defiance

Following rules and completing tasks can be trying experiences for children who have difficulty staying focused and achieving completion. In their efforts to avoid confusing or difficult situations, they may simply disregard what they are told. This can cause them to be seen as purposefully noncompliant, as though they are ignoring responsibility or being lazy. ADHD children with moderate to severe hyperactivity often yell, display aggression, or otherwise throw a tantrum when confronted for not following instructions. Those with little or no hyperactivity tend to verbally express their difficulties to some extent, although these attempts are often seen as excuses to be noncompliant.

### Impatience

Being patient can be difficult for the ADHD child. The days before a holiday or birthday can be particularly demanding. Waiting in line without an interesting focal point can seem unbearable, especially to children with severe hyperactivity, who may shove, hit, or cut in front of others who are ahead of them.

### Quick Frustration

The tolerance level of most ADHD children is very low. Failure to complete an effort after trying only once can cause the desire to give up.

### Anger

Due to their tendencies toward exaggerated emotions and quick frustration, ADHD children are prone to show anger easily. They generally become upset more quickly than other children, especially when teased or aggravated. The more hyperactive the child, the more likely he will be to show his frustration in the form of aggression.

### Forgetfulness

Many ADHD children have trouble remembering things. As their thoughts dart in different directions, they often lose sight of important dates, times, responsibilities, and opportunities. Ironically, however, some ADHD children have heightened memory capabilities.

### Disorganization

ADHD children tend to have messy bedrooms, backpacks, and desks. "Careless," "sloppy," and "lazy" are comments many of them hear regularly. They are frequently unable to find things, and often misplace important items. Homework and school papers are common examples. This lack of organization is directly related to forgetfulness and lack of focus.

## Social Displacement

ADHD children often have difficulty fitting in socially. They are frequently regarded as "different" or "immature," and tend to have problems dealing with their peers. Because an ADHD child's low frustration tolerance can be like a time bomb, relationships with others can become strained easily. Teasing and criticism can be intense, and as a result ADHD children may lie, argue and fight outwardly, while becoming depressed and anxious inwardly. In desperate attempts to control their social situations, some of these children are bossy, pushy, and intimidating. They often demand their own way and don't allow others to participate in activities. This is especially true of ADHD children with moderate to severe hyperactivity. As a result, many ADHD children choose to associate with those who are easily manipulated and/or younger.

## Insensitivity & Thoughtlessness

ADHD children may appear to have no regard for others' feelings, safety, and personal belongings, and may intrude on conversations and activities. The inappropriate actions these children display are usually unintentional. In many instances they are simply trying to get their message across before it becomes forgotten—overridden by other thoughts. They do not appear to realize the impact of their actions on others, and are often surprised by the negative responses they receive. When attempting to correct these behaviors, parents and teachers are often faced with an attitude of "I don't care," or told "It was his/her fault." Constantly attempting to derive attention, often by annoying means, is another hallmark of many ADHD children.

### Sleep Disturbances

Sleep patterns vary among those with ADHD. Some sleep lightly and show signs of restlessness, while others sleep quite deeply. Falling asleep at night may be a problem, even after an active day; however, these children will often fall asleep at impromptu times, such as during a short car ride.

### Coordination Difficulties

For some children, hyperactivity and inattention contribute to problems with coordination. Overactivity lends itself to clumsiness and poor foresight, while inattention causes a lack of focus on the task at hand. ADHD children also tend to have trouble balancing. This can make bike riding and other balance-oriented activities difficult or delayed for them. These children often have small or large muscle coordination deficiencies as well, although having problems in both muscle coordination groups is rare.

### Poor Verbalization & Expression

Some ADHD children have difficulty expressing themselves, and may stutter or forget what it is they are trying to say. Even when they do remember, presenting their thoughts in words may be slow, fast, or erratic and require a patient listener.

### Poor Perception & Application

ADHD children sometimes have difficulty under-standing directions in the form they are presented. As a result, they may need to hear or read directions more than once or have them presented in a variety of ways before they are able to carry out a task.

## Variations In Symptoms

The symptoms that constitute ADHD can vary greatly, with each child displaying his functional difficulties in a different way. While one child may exhibit a minimum of symptoms, another may have nearly all of them. In addition, each child's individual symptoms can range from mild to severe. For example, while one child might find sitting still almost impossible, another may have little or no trouble doing so. Finally, symptoms often fluctuate based on the circumstances a child is involved in at any given time. Assessing a child's symptoms can be a more difficult process for the parents of an only child who have little or no basis for comparison.

As this book progresses, drug-free ways to manage, improve, or eliminate ADHD symptoms will be explored. Practical suggestions on how to help ADHD children turn their difficulties into assets will also be presented. Keep in mind that variations of these ideas may be more beneficial for your child.

## Why Symptoms Aren't Enough For Diagnosis

Every child may, at one time or another, display the characteristics common to ADHD. Yet most children do not have ADHD. It is the frequency of symptoms and their level of interference with a child's ability to function that must be considered. A child whose attentional deficit is so great that he daydreams for the majority of each school day could obviously benefit from intervention. This child's consistent distraction would almost certainly affect his participation in class, as well as his ability to learn. On the other hand, a child who occasionally peers out the classroom window may be slightly distractible, although not enough to hinder his learning or otherwise cause him to be deemed inattentive.

The origin of symptoms must also be seriously considered. Among other things, medications, allergies, or medical problems may cause a child to appear as though he has ADHD when in fact he doesn't. Child abuse, depression, and other factors should be taken into account as well.

Age is another consideration. Very young children are naturally impulsive, inattentive, and overactive. These behaviors may be normal for them and therefore should not be considered symptoms of ADHD.

Overall, symptoms should be regarded as a tool in assessing a child's difficulties. They can further be used as a gauge in measuring levels of improvement.

# Chapter Two

## *Is It Really ADHD?*
### Identifying The Causes Of Hyperactivity & Inattention

Many children's struggles with hyperactivity and inattention are attributed to causes other than ADHD. Since drug therapy for ADHD can worsen certain conditions, or cause them to go undetected, it is essential that a child receive a complete and proper assessment considering all possible sources of difficulty before any type of medication is considered. This chapter presents a look at other possible causes of hyperactivity and inattention, and provides insight into how they may co-exist with, and affect, ADHD.

### *Physical Or Mental Illness*
Some forms of chronic illness can cause a child to show symptoms similar to those caused by ADHD. For example, a common trait of depression is lack of concentration—one of the main symptoms of inattention. Schizophrenia, autism, encephalitis, brain tumors, persistent headaches, and other problems can all present ADHD-like symptoms.

In some cases, ADHD may be present in conjunction with an existing illness. A number of children with underactive or overactive thyroid problems or seizure disorders also have ADHD. Additionally, nearly 70% of children with Tourette's syndrome are believed to have ADHD.

*Allergies*

An allergic reaction is the immune system's response to an offending substance. Such substances are called allergens. Allergens may be ingested, inhaled, or touched. Typical allergy symptoms include sneezing, runny nose, and itchy, watery eyes. Many people also experience itching and swelling of the mouth, throat, and inner ears; nausea or other stomach discomfort; and mild to severe skin rashes or hives. A child with allergies may have any combination of these symptoms. Resultingly, he may become frustrated, restless, irritable, and inattentive.

Constant or repeated contact with offending substances may make a child appear to have ADHD. Two of the most common food allergens, corn and peanuts, are often repeatedly fed to children in the form of corn flakes for breakfast and peanut butter sandwiches for lunch. Children who are allergic to these foods may have ongoing allergic reactions, causing a vicious circle of symptoms similar to ADHD. Constant contact allergens such as clothing soap or perfume may cause a similar effect.

Studies have shown that many children with allergies are hyperactive. Researchers have strived to find a causative relationship as to whether hyperactivity predisposes children to allergies, or whether allergies cause hyperactivity. In some cases, testing for allergies may be a worthwhile effort.

### Sensitivities

Sensitivities can appear in several different forms, including those related to food. Unlike food allergies, food sensitivities generally do not cause a reaction involving the immune system. Lactose intolerance, for example, is a sensitivity to dairy products; in effect it is a food sensitivity, rather than a food allergy. Other sensitivities include those related to touch, sound, smell, and sight. Each can cause its own particular difficulties.

In the case of touch sensitivities, or "tactile defensiveness," a child may repeatedly complain about irritation from clothing, the temperature of a room or bath water, and even the way his bed feels. Touch-sensitive children usually desire little or no physical contact with others, and may be averse to washing or otherwise touching themselves. They may routinely appear to be irritable and easily distracted.

A child who is distressed by many types of sound is said to be sound sensitive. Sounds that are too loud, too soft, or consistent can be particularly distracting and annoying. Children who are affected by this type of auditory disturbance may appear irritable, distracted, and emotional.

A child's sensitivity to smell can be baffling. While you may not recognize any particular scent, a smell-sensitive child may complain that a scent is overwhelming or makes him sick. This can cause a child to be irritable and distracted.

Children who are sight sensitive usually find sunlight, bright lights, flashing lights, and certain colors uncomfortable to look at. Some eye conditions and injuries can cause similar effects and therefore should be considered. A child who experiences sight sensitivity may appear emotional, irritable, and inattentive.

Each type of sensitivity can present symptoms similar to ADHD. In particular, the body's usual biochemical processes can be disturbed by sensitivities to food and smells. Children with more than one type of sensitivity may be "sensory defensive," and have several symptoms resembling ADHD. Children with sensitivities may also have ADHD.

### Yeast Overgrowth

An overabundance of the Candida albicans yeast in the body can cause thrush, rashes, and a variety of other physical problems. In addition, some doctors believe that yeast overgrowth is linked to various mental and central nervous system disturbances, including depression, autism, and hyperactivity. Antibiotics can encourage yeast overgrowth, especially with repeated use. ADHD may be present in conjunction with this condition.

### Inadequate Diet

Nutrition is essential to maintaining good health. Growing bodies constantly undergo change, making balanced nutrition important for proper development. Certain forms of nutrition are necessary for brain chemical regulation and aid in concentration (see chapter 8). An insufficient diet can cause a child to display a lack of concentration, inattentiveness, nervousness, or tiredness, or a combination of these. Some of the symptoms related to deficient nutrition may also resemble ADHD. Since many ADHD children crave sugar and sweets, they may be predisposed to poor nutrition. Therefore it is important to consider if ADHD and an inadequate diet are present together.

## Lack of Sleep

Insufficient sleep can cause a host of unpleasant symptoms, including poor concentration, emotionalism, hyperactivity, and irritability. Children who have chronic sleep problems (such as sleep apnea) or who obtain too little sleep on a regular basis may readily appear to have ADHD. Children with ADHD who do not get sufficient sleep usually have exaggerated symptoms.

## Child Abuse

Children who are physically, mentally, or sexually abused are often despondent and may appear inattentive, withdrawn, or emotional. Their symptoms may be a direct result of abuse; however, many abused children have ADHD to begin with. Their ADHD symptoms may cause or aggravate abuse situations.

### Substance Abuse

The effects of intentional drug misuse are many. A number of substances, both legal and illegal, can make a child without ADHD appear to have the condition.

### Hearing Problems

Children with distorted hearing or hearing loss often display inattentive and noncompliant behavior. Their auditory difficulties can cause them to lack focus and act frustrated, angry, and emotional. They may also have problems with verbalization and appear disorganized. Any of these actions may be incorrectly perceived as symptoms of ADHD.

Hearing problems can be caused by many factors, including ear canal blockage or inner ear injury (a ruptured eardrum, for example). Studies have shown a relationship between repeated ear infections and ADHD symptoms. It is important to rule out these possibilities before making a diagnosis of ADHD; however, keep in mind that a child with a hearing deficiency may have ADHD as well.

### Auditory Processing Difficulties

Children who have Central Auditory Processing Disorder (CAPD) or other problems related to the hearing-thought-action process may be distractible, frustrated, restless, irritable, and emotional. ADHD may also be present in these children.

## Visual Impairments

Poor vision and sight disturbances such as near-sightedness or farsightedness often cause children to become restless, frustrated, and irritable. A child who cannot see correctly may also become withdrawn or highly emotional. It is important to remember that school-issued vision tests are conducted only once each year, and a child's vision may deteriorate *after* testing.

Eyeglasses that are too tight or have incorrect prescriptions; dry eyes (due to contact lenses, medications or other causes); and reactions to eye drops can cause visual discomfort and disturbances. Conditions such as lazy eye, in which the eye's muscular system is underdeveloped or has otherwise been weakened, can also be troublesome. Although ADHD may also be present, vision problems should always be considered.

## Visual Processing Deficits

Difficulty retaining and using perceptually-derived information (such as being unable to copy a word or image from a blackboard to paper) can cause frustration, restlessness, irritability, and emotionalism. ADHD may exist concurrently.

## Sensory Integration Deficits

Children who have difficulty processing information through their sensory channels (especially sight, hearing, and touch) may have a majority of the symptoms common to ADHD. Studies have suggested that some children with sensory integration deficits also have ADHD.

## Anxiety & Related Disorders

Lack of attention, constant distractibility, and excessive drive are characteristic of anxiety. Related disorders include separation-anxiety disorder, overanxious disorder, and post-traumatic stress disorder. Since anxiety symptoms so closely resemble ADHD, careful observation and assessment are needed for an accurate diagnosis. In some cases, anxiety and ADHD are present together.

## Effects Of Medication

Many medications can cause hyperactivity or inattention. For example, cold and allergy drugs which contain ephedrine and pseudoephedrine can make children restless and anxious, while medications used to control seizures and convulsions (such as phenobarbital and phenytoin) can cause children to be tired, irritable, and inattentive. ADHD may be present in addition to symptoms induced by medication.

## Metal Intoxication

Studies show that high levels of metal in the bloodstream can cause distortions in behavior. Lead, found in the paint, household dust, and surrounding soil of millions of old homes and in many antiques (including painted wooden toys), is a highly toxic substance known to cause hyperactivity and other neurological disturbances. Lead has also been found in water which has traveled through plumbing pipes repaired with lead-based solder.

Mercury toxicity also causes behavior-related problems in children. These include hyperactivity, depression, and irritability. Mercury is found in fish, shellfish, fabric softeners, plastics, certain inks and paints, and dental fillings. It is more toxic than lead.

Copper overexposure in children is another form of metal intoxication. Improper copper metabolism in the body, in which excess absorption occurs, is a condition called Wilson's disease. Although relatively rare, this congenital disorder is characterized by an overload of copper accumulating in the brain and other areas of the body. Irritability, confusion, and other behavior-related problems often result.

Although not a heavy metal like lead or copper, aluminum is also toxic. It is frequently found in cookware, utensils, baking soda, flour, cake mixes, pancake and biscuit mixes, processed cheese, antiperspirants, over-the-counter medications, various tap water sources, and several forms of packaging, including cans. Excessive antacid intake is the most commonly reported form of aluminum toxicity. Symptoms include severe nervousness, forgetfulness, memory loss, and speech distortions.

With the exception of Wilson's disease, the risk of metal intoxication in children can be greatly reduced by avoiding the sources of toxicity. Parents whose occupations or hobbies require them to work with metals, such as welders, can further protect their children by keeping tools and work clothes (especially after use) out of reach.

It is possible for a child with metal intoxication to have ADHD as well. A hair analysis can confirm or rule out metal intoxication.

### Learning Disabilities

Difficulties in perception, expression, integration, and memorization are the basis of many learning inabilities. Perception-related learning disabilities are those in which a child has difficulty differentiating between visual (sight-related) or auditory (hearing-related) situations. For example, a child with an auditory deficit may have trouble identifying differences in sound. As a result, he may lag behind others in properly vocalizing the letters of the alphabet.

Expression disabilities are those that relate to communication. A child with language difficulties may find reading and writing extremely challenging. Coordination and motor difficulties can also cause problems with verbalization and writing.

A child who experiences difficulty organizing his thoughts and utilizing the information he hears or reads may suffer from an integration-related learning disability. This child may be unable to follow directions and become frustrated with simple tasks.

Similar to a child with an integration disability, a child with a memory disability may be unable to follow through with directions. The inability to "store" collected information, even for short periods of time, can make all forms of verbal and written communication strenuous.

Each type of learning disability presents its own problems and can make a child feel embarrassed, frustrated, irritable, withdrawn, emotional, and inattentive. Since many children who have learning disabilities also have ADHD, it may be difficult to recognize which symptoms are related to which problem. Carefully assessing each symptom individually may be helpful.

## Head Injuries

Severe head trauma resulting in bruised brain tissue, brain stem damage, or skull fracture may cause several neurologically-related symptoms including poor memory, distractibility, and inattentiveness. A child with ADHD who sustains such an injury is likely to have intensified symptoms.

## Diabetes & Hypoglycemia

Disturbances in the regulation of insulin within the body can cause several symptoms common to ADHD. Diabetes, the result of insufficient insulin production by the pancreas, leaves the body unable to properly utilize glucose (blood sugar). Juvenile, or Type I diabetes, is known to produce irritability, weakness, and fatigue, among other symptoms. It is estimated that over 10 million people in the U.S.—many of which are children—have diabetes.

Hypoglycemia, or low blood sugar, is the result of an overabundance of insulin being produced by the pancreas. Irritability, nervousness, anxiety, confusion, depression, dizziness, and fatigue are among the symptoms that characterize this disorder. Diet plays a major role in eliminating symptoms. Hypoglycemia may be hereditary or the result of a consistently poor diet. ADHD can be present in addition to either hypoglycemia or diabetes.

### Stress

Stress can cause many physical and mental symptoms. Severe stress may be caused by divorce, a death, or a major relocation, among other things. Situation-related stresses caused by being exposed to repetitive uncomfortable conditions may produce mild, moderate, or severe stress. A chaotic home life is a good example. Since stress is perceived differently by everyone, children with mild to extreme stress may appear withdrawn, inattentive, fidgety, depressed, angry, or emotional. Not only can ADHD be present in addition to stress, it may also be the cause of it.

### Forced Pre-development

Forced premature development, in which a parent or caretaker consistently requires a child to perform well above his age level, can cause a child to be irritable, impatient, nervous, angry, and depressed. Constant inappropriate expectations and unrealistic demands imposed on a child may make him appear to have ADHD.

Many children with ADHD are highly intelligent. Unfortunately, their intelligence may predispose them to either intentional or unintentional forced pre-development. This is likely to increase ADHD symptoms in affected children.

### Behavioral Disorders

Behavioral conditions unrelated to hyperactivity and inattention may exist alone or in addition to ADHD. Conduct Disorder and Oppositional Defiant Disorder are the most common examples.

Conduct Disorder (CD) is characterized mainly by deliberate and destructive behaviors such as dishonesty, theft, drug abuse, truancy, vandalism, and fighting. Rare in young children, this disorder is generally more prevalent in those approaching adolescence.

Oppositional Defiant Disorder (ODD) is identified by a consistent negative attitude and mood, as well as aggressiveness and inconsideration. Unlike Conduct Disorder, it is common before adolescence.

Since both of these disorders can cause a child to appear aggressive, impulsive, and uncooperative, they may be mistaken for ADHD. The presence of ADHD in addition to a behavioral disorder is a valid possibility and should be considered.

## Other Considerations

There are many other possible causes of ADHD symptoms. Loud, overcrowded classrooms, for example, can provide more stimuli than some children can—or care to—handle. As a result, a child may "act out" and appear to have ADHD, when in fact he may be showing his frustration at being unable to function at his best under the given conditions.

Another consideration is that children, like adults, have their "peak" times. Some children are most attentive and productive first thing in the morning, while others are at their best after lunch, after school, or in the evening.

Although this list provides insight into many possible causes of ADHD-type symptoms, there are others. All factors should be considered before confirming or accepting a diagnosis of ADHD or agreeing to drug therapy.

# Chapter Three

## *Avoiding Drug Therapy*
### Insight & Perspectives

It is estimated that in nearly fifty percent of all visits to doctors for problems related to hyperactivity and attention deficits, medication is prescribed. This high ratio has many factors behind it, some of which are unfortunately not in a child's best interests. A frequent example can be seen in situations with overburdened teachers and parents. A teacher whose class size and job requirements are excessive is likely to become easily frustrated by a child's repeated acting out or lack of focus. Parents who work long hours and have numerous responsibilities are also apt to become easily frustrated by a child who exhibits these behaviors. Constant notes and phone calls from a frazzled teacher to overwhelmed parents often result in a visit to the child's doctor—and a request for medication. In this scenario, a child may end up being medicated mainly for the convenience of the parents and teacher.

Although improper, teachers often outright recommend that parents have their child medicated. Some even suggest a particular medication and dosage. A teacher should never make these recommendations.

Teachers rarely know the entire medical history of a child, and it is unlikely that they are trained to make a complete assessment of the root of the child's difficulties. This is not to say, however, that a teacher's mention of a child's problems should not be acknowledged and seriously investigated. A teacher's observations can be a useful tool in alerting parents and in helping a physician to make a clearer assessment and more accurate diagnosis. A teacher's efforts can also play a major role in helping a child toward improvement, regardless of the cause of his difficulties.

Frighteningly, some doctors prescribe medication for ADHD-type symptoms by phone at the request of parents and teachers. This can cause a host of additional problems. Even when teachers and parents feel they are making an accurate analysis of a child's problems, and a doctor is familiar with the child, every other possibility needs to be explored. Before medication is considered a child should receive a thorough physical in which sight, hearing, blood pressure, blood sugar levels, and other important medical aspects are checked. A review of the child's diet and sleep habits is also essential.

A child should also be directly "interviewed" by one or more doctors. By asking questions regarding a child's physical and mental health, lifestyle, and habits, a physician may be able to detect a cause of hyperactivity or attention deficits other than ADHD. In many instances it is found that a child does not have ADHD at all. However, if a child still appears to have ADHD after all other possibilities have been exhausted, the next step is to decide on a treatment program.

## Saying No To Drug Therapy

The decision to avoid drug therapy as a means of treatment for hyperactivity and attention deficits may be due to necessity or choice. Listed here are some of the more common reasons why drug therapy is likely to require avoidance:

### Allergy To Medication
An obvious allergic reaction to a medication, such as hives or breathing difficulties, most often indicates that it should not be used.

### Sensitivity To Medication
Constant uncomfortable effects, including fever and skin rashes, may indicate a sensitivity that warrants not taking a particular drug.

### Drug Interactions
Improper combinations of medication can result in the ineffectiveness of one or more drugs, or a serious reaction. Antihistamines, antidepressants, and blood pressure medications are among the drugs that should not be combined with those commonly prescribed for the treatment of ADHD.

*Anxiety*

A number of medications used to treat ADHD can produce or increase anxiousness and nervousness, therefore causing a child who already has anxiety problems to feel these symptoms at intense levels. Consequently, drug therapy is generally avoided in children with anxiety disorders.

*Psychosis*

Psychotic episodes tend to be worsened by many medications used for ADHD treatment. As a result, several drugs used to treat ADHD are usually not prescribed for those who suffer from psychosis.

*Tics*

Children who have a tic disorder or Tourette's syndrome may be unable to receive drug therapy for ADHD due to the possibility of medication worsening the tics. Although some doctors prescribe major tranquilizers along with stimulants in an attempt to simultaneously control both ADHD symptoms and the involuntary muscle reactions of tics, there is concern about the possible risks with this type of dual medicating. A family history of tic disorder or Tourette's syndrome may be an indicator that medication for ADHD should be avoided.

*High Blood Pressure*

Medication for ADHD may increase blood pressure, reduce the effect of blood pressure medication, or both. Alternate forms of therapy are often chosen for those who have hypertension.

### Glaucoma

Certain forms of this disease, characterized by unusually high fluid pressure in the eye and possible loss of sight, may be worsened by medications prescribed for ADHD. As a result, drug therapy for ADHD is often bypassed as a treatment option for those with glaucoma.

### Hyperthyroidism

This condition causes elevated blood pressure and heart rate. Certain drugs prescribed for ADHD can also produce these effects, making a potentially dangerous combination. Other types of therapy are generally recommended.

### Liver Disease

Several medications used to treat ADHD can adversely affect liver function and therefore should be avoided in those with liver disease.

### Cardiovascular Disease

Due to their tendency to increase blood pressure and heart rate, most medications recommended for ADHD are not considered in the treatment of children with cardiovascular disease and related conditions.

### Seizure Disorders

Stimulant medications prescribed for ADHD may increase the frequency of seizures. Some doctors prescribe anticonvulsants together with stimulants in the hopes of improving ADHD symptoms without increasing the possibility of seizures. However, since anticonvulsant medications can also cause ADHD-like symptoms, avoidance is often preferable.

### Growth Suppression

Children whose growth rates are reduced due to sleep apnea are likely to experience further difficulty in both sleeping and eating when administered stimulant medication. Rectifying the cause of the sleep disorder—which may in itself be the cause of ADHD-type symptoms—is often the best alternative.

### Eating Disorders

Several drugs prescribed for ADHD, including Ritalin and Prozac, can cause a lack of appetite. These medications are often avoided in the treatment of children with eating disorders.

## Avoiding Drug Therapy By Choice

Many parents whose children are not restricted from utilizing drug therapy choose to avoid it for other reasons. Several of these reasons are listed in the pages that follow.

## Risk Of Side Effects

The possibility of adverse effects is one of the major reasons parents oppose drug therapy for their hyperactive and inattentive children. The decision to avoid medication can be further promoted by a family history of health problems, especially when a child is in a high-risk category.

## Age

Parents often decide against drug therapy due to a child's age. For example, many parents of young children have concerns about the effects of medication on a child's development. Parents of teenagers are often opposed to drug therapy due to the potential for abuse. Resistance to take medication for social reasons can also be a factor with adolescents.

## Inconvenience

Monitoring medication times can be tedious, especially when a regimen must be set up both at home and at school. Parents sometimes avoid drug therapy for their children as a result.

## Embarrassment

While many children with ADHD show a lack of conscience concerning actions that affect others, they often have exaggerated inward emotions. As a result, they may feel extremely embarrassed about taking medication. Parents may also feel some degree of embarrassment at the prospect of medicating their child. Drug therapy may be better off avoided in these situations.

### Attitude

Children who are determined to make improvements without drug therapy are often successful. Most parents are eager to try other forms of intervention when a child has a positive attitude.

### Child's Mental Health

Parents who feel a child's concern over taking medication will cause him excessive stress often forego drug therapy and utilize other treatment options.

### Insufficient Drug Studies

A lack of conclusive evidence regarding the effects of long-term use makes many parents wary of drugs prescribed for ADHD. It has recently been suggested that long-term use of stimulants may worsen ADHD symptoms once medication has been stopped. There has also been concern over whether stimulant therapy can permanently alter brain chemistry.

### Addiction Potential

Several medications prescribed for ADHD can be addictive. As a result, many parents—especially those whose ADHD children are adolescents—opt for other forms of treatment.

## Forced Drug Therapy

Forced drug therapy is an area of much controversy. There are two types. The first is parent or caretaker-induced, caused by demanding that a child take medication for ADHD-type behaviors regardless of his objections or physical discomfort from side effects. This may actually cause a child to suffer additional—and possibly more serious—problems both physically and mentally. Spousal pressure, in which one parent demands that a child be medicated against the other's better judgement, can be a factor in this type of situation.

The second type of forced drug therapy involves schooling. Various educational districts have sought court orders to require that parents medicate their children during school hours. This has opened up many new areas of argument and has met with much resistance.

Children should not be forced to take medication, and parents should not have to medicate their children against their will. The negative impact of demanding the use of medication can be quite destructive. Respect, honesty, and understanding—the building blocks for every successful relationship in life—can be severely affected or destroyed by forcing a child to take medication. Parents who are forced to medicate their children generally feel resentment, anger, guilt, embarrassment, and other feelings which are not conducive to helping an ADHD child toward improvement of his difficulties.

## Commonly Prescribed Drugs

Medications regularly prescribed for ADHD symptoms and behaviors include stimulants, tranquilizers, and antidepressants. Of these, stimulants are the most commonly used. Other medications, such as tricyclic antidepressants (also referred to as TCAs) or tranquilizers are often used when stimulants cause problematic effects or prove to be ineffective. Each of these medications has associated health risks. Several of the drugs currently used to treat ADHD are described in the following pages.

### *Stimulants*

### RITALIN
Ritalin is the commonly known brand name for methylphenidate. This drug was first introduced into the medical community in 1960. Currently available in tablet form, Ritalin is the most frequently prescribed medication for ADHD and related behavioral disorders. It is estimated that nearly two million children in the country are presently taking the drug.

Extensive controversy surrounds Ritalin use, with advocates desperately trying to promote the drug as "safe" and those opposed to its use adamantly proclaiming it as "dangerous." Lawsuits and spurts of negative and positive media coverage over the years have inevitably caused an ebb and flow effect in sales of the drug. However, current usage continues to grow.

According to CIBA Pharmaceutical Company, makers of Ritalin, the drug is "a mild central nervous system stimulant." Although research has yet to confirm exactly how Ritalin works, it is assumed to affect the brain stem arousal system and cortex—areas within the central nervous system.

Possible side effects of Ritalin include nervousness, sleeplessness, drowsiness, hypersensitivity, loss of appetite, anorexia, abdominal pain, weight loss, headache, nausea, dizziness, variations in pulse and blood pressure, dyskinesia (movement disturbances), and heart-related effects such as palpitations, tachycardia, angina, and cardiac arrhythmia. Toxic psychosis may also occur. The most common effects children experience are loss of appetite, weight loss, abdominal pain, sleeplessness, and tachycardia. Mood changes are also frequently reported.

Ritalin reduces the effectiveness of guanethidine, a medication prescribed for high blood pressure. Taken together with monoamine oxidase (MAO) inhibitors, the effect of Ritalin may increase to dangerous levels. Interaction with anticonvulsant drugs, anti-coagulants (blood-thinning medications), antidepressants, or anti-inflammatory medications such as phenylbutazone may cause these drugs to break down slowly in the body and remain in the bloodstream for longer periods of time.

The drug insert for Ritalin specifically states that it should not be used in children under the age of six, as safety and efficacy of the drug have not been established in this age group. The insert also warns that the safety of long-term use of the drug has not been established, as sufficient data is not yet available. Further, it is recommended that treatment with Ritalin include a combined program of psychological, behavioral, educational, and social intervention and assistance. Family and group therapy is often suggested as part of treatment; however, some reports indicate that a high percentage of children who take the drug receive little or no counseling or intervention.

## CYLERT

Cylert is the brand name for pemoline. Like Ritalin, this psychotherapeutic drug stimulates the central nervous system. While Ritalin's effectiveness generally lasts between three and four hours, Cylert appears to remain effective for approximately seven. About one percent of children treated with Cylert experience a severe sensitivity to the drug which affects the liver and can be dangerous. Consequently, children for whom Cylert is prescribed should be closely medically monitored.

## DEXEDRINE

Dexedrine, Oxydess, and Spancap are brand names for dextroamphetamine (also referred to as d-amphetamine). This stimulant drug is highly addictive and usage must be carefully regulated. The use of a monoamine oxidase (MAO) inhibitor with dextro-amphetamine can cause a severe drop in blood pressure. Dextroamphetamine and MAO inhibitors should not be taken within 14-21 days of each other. Drug therapy with dextroamphetamine should be avoided for children with high blood pressure, thyroid problems, heart disease, and glaucoma, and carefully regulated in those taking insulin.

## Antidepressants

### ELAVIL

Elavil is the brand name for amitriptyline, also known under the brand name Endep. It is used to treat depression with or without anxiety. This drug has an extensive list of possible side effects, including excitement and restlessness—the same symptoms common to hyperactivity. Taken together with Ritalin, Elavil is retained in the body for a longer period of time and may cause overdosage.

### AVENTYL

Aventyl and Pamelor are brand names for the drug nortriptyline. This drug's effects are quite similar to Elavil, including the possible risk of overdose when combined with Ritalin.

### TOFRANIL

Tofranil, Tofranil-PM, and Janimine are the trade

names for imipramine. Like Elavil and Aventyl, Tofranil is used to alleviate depression and related anxiety, and should not be combined with Ritalin. Taken with an MAO inhibitor, imipramine can cause convulsions or death.

## PROZAC

Known to most people as Prozac, fluoxetine hydrochloride has a chemical makeup which is different from other antidepressants. This drug may improve mental alertness; however, its possible side effects are numerous. Some physicians prescribe Prozac together with Ritalin for the treatment of ADHD. Both of these drugs can cause weight loss and may affect growth and development. Prozac remains in the body for a number of weeks after discontinuation of the drug. Its possible side effects include anxiety, nervousness, and lack of concentration.

## NORPRAMIN

Norpramin and Pertofrane are known brand names for the drug desipramine. This medication is an antidepressant generally used to treat depression with or without anxiety. It is not recommended for use in children. Although some doctors feel desipramine is more effective than Ritalin and has less side effects, its potential side effects include many of the same symptoms as ADHD itself. In addition, this drug's history includes the sudden deaths of a number of children being treated with it for hyperactivity.

## WELLBUTRIN

Wellbutrin is the brand name for bupropion hydrochloride. Generally prescribed for mild depression, this drug's chemical makeup is similar to the appetite suppressant diethylpropion. Bupropion carries a high seizure risk and an abundance of other potential side effects, including aggressiveness, restlessness, anxiety, agitation, insomnia, sight and hearing disturbances, and loss of concentration. In addition, this drug can cause appetite disturbances and weight loss, and may cause a child to feel "high." Hallucinations and psychotic episodes have been reported during use. Children with seizure disorders, heart disease, liver disease, and other medical problems should not take bupropion. This drug's side effects can be so severe that approximately 1 out of every 10 people for whom it is prescribed cease taking it.

### Tranquilizers

## VALIUM

Valium is the well-known brand name for diazepam. Other brand names for diazepam are Valrelease and Zetran. This drug is a minor tranquilizer generally prescribed to reduce anxiety, prevent convulsions, or promote sleep; however, it is sometimes prescribed for hyperactivity as well. Like other tranquilizers, Valium can cause impaired concentration, and as a result may aggravate inattentiveness.

## LIBRIUM

Librium, Libritabs, Mitran, and Reposans-10 are brand names for chlordiazepoxide. Similar to Valium, Librium is a minor tranquilizer. This drug can cause drowsiness, confusion, depression, and nervousness in addition to other symptoms. Among other drugs, MAO inhibitors and antihistamines should be avoided while taking chlordiazepoxide.

## VISTARIL

Vistaril, Hydroxyzine Pamoate, Hydroxyzine Hydrochloride, Anxanil, and Atarax are all brand names for hydroxyzine. Interestingly, this drug is an antihistamine used not only for the effects of allergies, but also for anxiety, agitation, and hyperactivity. Hydroxyzine should not be combined with other antihistamines.

## Other Medications

Lithium, a drug commonly used to treat manic depression (also known as bipolar disorder); Clonidine, generally used to treat high blood pressure; Haldol, prescribed mainly for psychotic disorders; and Tegretol, an anticonvulsant drug, have also been known to be prescribed for the symptoms characteristic to ADHD. Clonidine or Haldol are sometimes prescribed for children with ADHD and Tourette's syndrome; however, these drugs are not effective for every symptom of ADHD and carry the possibility of worsening the tics.

Current experimental medications include the weight-control drug Pondimin and a high blood pressure medicine known as Inderal. Each of these medications carries its own contraindications and risks. There are no extensive studies on how these drugs affect ADHD.

## The Benefits Of Avoidance

Every so often a parent will be heard saying how "miraculous" drug therapy for ADHD is. "My kid is a different person," "I wish I'd done this sooner," and "I don't know how my family survived before my child started taking medication" are frequent comments. But again, in whose best interest is a child being medicated? Furthermore, what kind of effect will be made on children who come to believe that they need a pill to be more in control, more social, and more accepted by their families? Finally, are the children for which drug therapy is contraindicated or ineffective to believe that there is no hope for improving *their* symptoms?

Drug therapy is not a miracle cure for ADHD. Not unlike taking medication for pain, it is simply a way to temporarily control symptoms. And there are options. Other methods may take more effort; they may not provide the "quick relief" afforded by some medications. But their long-term effects can be very worthwhile. The effort expended can provide a more solid foundation in many aspects of a child's life. Learning to compensate for difficulties early on can help children progress in life without using drugs as a crutch.

In this age of fast living, it is tempting to find the quickest remedy to a problem. It is important not to forget the all-important adage that nothing good comes easy.

While most doctors will suggest a multimodal treatment approach including medication, there are many cases in which behavioral modification, proper educational placement, and other forms of drug-free intervention can be just as effective. This can be especially true with cases of mild to moderate ADHD. Even in cases of severe ADHD, children can be taught skills to improve their symptoms and behaviors. The key is to find the most effective form of drug-free treatment for each particular child and combine it with tireless patience and understanding.

Some will argue that this approach takes too much time, doesn't gain support from teachers, denies siblings of needed attention, and drains parents of energy. But by making strides in the right direction—even through the slowest progress—these situations can improve or even be eliminated. The added effort can also result in appreciation and respect from the child.

There are several benefits to avoiding drug therapy. Those that follow are only a few of the more universal examples. Each child and family may have their own reasons why avoidance is beneficial.

## No Drug Side Effects

If a child is not being medicated for ADHD, he can avoid suffering from drug-induced effects. These include "rebound," a common side effect in which behavior-related symptoms actually become worse than normal as medication begins to wear off.

## No Drug Tolerance Concerns

There are no worries over a medication becoming ineffective when drug-free intervention is used.

## No Inconvenience

Without drug therapy, there is no need to remember medication times, bring medication along, or refill prescriptions.

## No Embarrassment

There is no possibility of becoming embarrassed about drug therapy when medication is not being used. Adolescents are often particularly sensitive in this area.

## No Worry Of Shortage

Drug shortages, such as the Ritalin shortage in 1993, are of no concern when medication is not part of a treatment plan. There is no need to search for a drug at numerous pharmacies, and no worry about how a child will fare without medication.

### No Cost To Medicate

The monies saved on prescriptions and doctor visits for ADHD can effectively be used toward other forms of intervention.

### No Withdrawal Symptoms

Depression, sleeplessness, rebound, and other symptoms caused by withdrawal are avoided when drug therapy is not used.

### Enhanced Pride & Accomplishment

Feelings of accomplishment from developing better skills of self-control without drugs can build a child's self-esteem in many ways. The pride that results can instill a "can do" attitude and the will to continue making improvements. Many parents feel that the skills their children build in this manner are more valued than those they are able to master while medicated. These skills can benefit a child throughout his teenage years and into adulthood.

## Alternative Treatments

Concern over the safety of current medical treatment available for ADHD prompts many parents to consider other options. However, there is much disagreement over whether certain treatments and interventions can actually improve or eliminate the symptoms of ADHD. The fact is, each child may respond differently to different forms of therapy.

What may prove to be ineffective for one child may in fact be beneficial for another.

The key to trying alternative treatments is to keep a reasonable perspective and not expect immediate improvement. Most importantly, try only those therapies which seem reasonable and harmless. Beware of unproven treatments that are dangerous or costly.

A significant number of parents have reported vast improvements in their ADHD children by combining alternative therapies. One such combination is dietary modification (see chapter 8) and physical exercise. Studies have shown that both of these interventions can promote relaxation and attentiveness in hyperactive children. Be sure to consult a physician regarding a child's diet and exercise habits before making any changes.

A percentage of parents with concerns over the numerous possible side effects of popular drug therapies have successfully used the amino acid known as GABA (gamma-amino butyric acid) or the herb valerian root in treating ADHD symptoms. Studies have shown that GABA can lessen hyperactivity and reduces the tendency toward learning disabilities. According to medical experts, there is no risk of addiction to GABA.

Valerian root has long been used as a calming agent by those who have difficulty falling asleep. Currently, many parents are using this herb for the treatment of hyperactivity. There are no reported side effects.

## Adolescents And Medication

Doctors and parents are often hesitant to use stimulant therapy for teenagers. This reluctancy is a result of several factors, including the very real possibility of abuse and addiction. Reports of adolescents crushing and inhaling stimulants, exceeding oral doses, and selling their medication to others have caused concern for parents and doctors alike.

Those teenagers who take medication responsibly are likely to face other issues. Many adolescents do not want to take medication for a number of personal and social reasons. Forcing them to do so may create resentment, while allowing them to regulate their own medication can result in none being taken.

Drug therapy and driving is another area of concern and controversy that surrounds teenagers with ADHD. Some parents feel their ADHD adolescents should be medicated to drive in order to maintain focus. Others worry that the medication may cause "overfocus," restricting a teenager from envisioning the "whole picture" and driving defensively.

## In Conclusion

When deciding upon a treatment plan, it is important to remember that the effort invested into a child's overall well-being benefits not only the child, but also his family and society as a whole. Although in some cases it may be felt that drug therapy is a useful or necessary adjunct in gaining control of symptoms, maintaining that control without medication is a worthwhile goal.

# Chapter Four

## *Attitude & Capability*
### Utilizing The Benefits Of Self-Esteem

Children who possess feelings of self-worth and have belief in their abilities are able to experience the advantages of having high self-esteem. Their confident attitudes help them readily establish goals, fit in with peers, and overcome obstacles. Their triumphs lead to a better outlook on life.

ADHD children often miss out on these benefits. Because they tend to be repeatedly reprimanded, humiliated, teased, and misunderstood, their strengths and talents frequently go unnoticed. Further, their true levels of intelligence are often unrecognized and highly underutilized. Many of these children become ashamed of themselves and their actions, and believe that no one likes them. As a result of their inability to feel important, capable, and accepted, they often acquire poor self-images.

Improving the self-esteem of ADHD children is essential in helping them to minimize their difficulties. It can also help to eliminate the need for medication. Self-esteem can be developed by focusing on a child's talents and strengths, and maintained by lessening rejections and failures. Parents and teachers can help by promoting positive feelings, giving encouragement, and providing opportunities for goals that can be accomplished. This chapter takes a look at the areas where self-esteem is most affected, and offers useful suggestions on how to help ADHD children develop lasting feelings of positive self-worth.

## Acknowledging A Child's Difficulties

The way in which a child is approached about his problems can have a great impact on self-esteem. Many doctors and mental health professionals believe that the best way to start treatment with an ADHD child is to tell him straight out what is causing his difficulties. But how do parents and doctors best explain what ADHD is when no one really knows what causes it? Further, how do they effectively make children understand that having a brain-related problem doesn't mean a person is "crazy" or "mental"? Lastly, how are children to distinguish between difficulties related to ADHD and those that are normal? While some children may find relief in knowing that there is a possible cause for some of the difficulties they face, the long-term effect of being told they have a problem with their brain could in fact be disastrous to self-esteem.

By telling a child he has an "incurable" disorder he is likely to feel defeated from the start. By stating that he has difficulties which can be improved upon, you give the child hope and the will to try, rather than disassembling his self-esteem. Helping a child forge ahead toward solutions to his difficulties (or at least effective management of them) may be easier to do if the child is not mentally laden with the idea that he has a disorder.

Some will argue that this approach can set a child up for failure, stating that if the child does not see a vast improvement in his difficulties right away, he is likely to give up. But it must be remembered that the only failure is in not trying, and that by consistently encouraging a child and applauding his efforts you can greatly improve his chances for success. It should be emphasized to a child that improvement takes time.

## Enabling vs. Labeling

Labeling a child as ADHD may cause others to believe that he has all of the symptoms or behavioral difficulties characteristic of ADHD, when in fact it is rare to find a child who has even a majority of them. Labeling can also increase the likelihood of a child being omitted or removed from activities he enjoys and does well at. It can also set him up for added teasing and humiliation.

Acknowledging and addressing a child's problems can be done without labeling. You can still let a child know that you are aware of his difficulties and that you care. Also consider that if a child hears or sees information on ADHD—which is becoming a common topic—he will be unlikely to become worried or frightened by what is said or written. Most of all it is important to remember that the same management techniques can be applied without a label that are applied with one.

There is also no real need to label a child at school. There is simply a need for his teacher to be aware of his difficulties and help him improve upon them. Even with severe cases of ADHD, or in cases where a child attends special classes, labeling is unnecessary. Due to the fact that each child may have a different set of problems, avoiding a label and concentrating on individual difficulties can prove more effective and successful. This is not unlike describing the symptoms of a cold to a doctor. You might have a congested nose, scratchy throat, and dry cough. Or you might have a runny nose, a sore throat, and no cough. Either way you may have a cold. But in order to prescribe effectively and help you to improve, the doctor needs to concentrate on your exact symptoms. The same concept applies with ADHD.

Parents sometimes use the label of ADHD to relieve guilt when they realize their child's difficulties are not due to inadequate parenting. Some also use it as a diagnosis for insurance reimbursement purposes, and even as a tax deduction by listing their child as "handicapped." But again, it is important to assess whether any of these actions will benefit a child's self-esteem.

## Telling Others

By alerting new teachers to a child's difficulties (without labeling), parents may be able to fend off problems before they start. This is best done at the beginning of the school year. There are parents, however, who do not agree with this idea. These parents contend that a child should get a "fair shake" with new teachers and classmates, and should not be "tagged as trouble" from the onset. However, alerting teachers to a child's problem areas at the start can be a win-win situation. It shows teachers that you are an involved and caring parent, and allows them to implement helpful strategies (such as seating placement) for your child. In the event a child progresses without difficulty, parents can feel proud and appreciative that their child is doing well. If the child begins to have difficulty, his teacher may be better prepared to provide him with assistance.

Another area of telling others involves siblings. Some people contend that siblings should be taken aside and privately told of their brother or sister's "problem." Given that children can be quite cruel during arguments, this confidential information may be seen as the perfect "ammunition" to hurt another. Others insist that a family should sit down as a group and discuss an ADHD child's problems. This may also be defeating to the child and may encourage him to use his problems as an excuse in different situations. Not making an issue out of a child's difficulties may be the least destructive way to handle the situation. Continually reinforcing the idea that everyone learns at their own pace and that each person may handle a situation differently will not only prompt siblings to respect the differences of an ADHD brother or sister, but also the differences of others they will encounter throughout their lives.

## Medication & Self-Esteem

While medication may help control various symptoms of ADHD and allow children the opportunity to experience positive interactions, it can actually cause lower self-esteem in the long run if a child believes he cannot "function properly" or act "normal" without it. Also, when parents applaud medication—rather than their child—for changes that take place during drug therapy, they can make him feel depressed and inferior. Children who are required to take more than one drug (such as those taking stimulants who need additional medication to fall asleep) may feel these emotions in greater impact. Other forms of therapy can eliminate this risk.

## Self-Esteem & School

School presents many opportunities for a child's self-esteem to be affected. ADHD children are particularly prone to assaults on self-esteem because they are often seen as "different" from their peers. Many get caught up in a continual cycle of negative comments and teasing from other students and abrasive treatment from teachers. Several studies on children in classroom settings have shown that teachers issue more negative feedback and harsher discipline to ADHD students than to other students. These situations can cause a child to develop a low self-image, and can increase feelings of sadness and worthlessness.

Parents and teachers need to take steps to protect and enhance the self-esteem of ADHD children at school. Parents can help by making sure that their children do not stand out from their peers in appearance and hygiene. They can also help by teaching their children appropriate social skills.

Teachers can help by realizing the impact of certain actions and avoiding them. For example, a teacher who recognizes the negative effect of alerting an entire class to a child's areas of needed improvement might inform the child individually. Thereby the teacher can help the child preserve his dignity. Teachers can further assist ADHD children in maintaining and improving self-esteem in the following ways:

- Avoid singling out an ADHD child, unless to give praise.
- Display all childrens' work, not only those who do the best work.
- Emphasize an ADHD child's strengths.
- Encourage other students to respect an ADHD child's differences.

- Provide an ADHD child with goals he can readily accomplish.
- Listen to and acknowledge an ADHD child's concerns and suggestions.
- Acknowledge mistakes and give encouragement.
- Enforce disciplinary actions without disrespect.
- Avoid insulting or embarrassing a child.

## Improving Attitude

An ADHD child's attitude may be a reflection of frustration and anger, or self-pity and depression. He may be negative, or simply complacent and uncaring. Repeated attacks on self-esteem can cause a child with ADHD (or any other child, for that matter) to become withdrawn and block out whatever disturbs him. This type of continual no-emotion "conditioning" does not allow self-esteem to be nurtured and grow. All of the child's energies are tied up in constantly blocking out negative feedback. In order to begin building self-esteem and gain a better attitude, this type of cycle must be broken.

Assessing a child's attitude is the first step toward helping him gain a more positive outlook. From there, a plan should be devised to help the child build self-esteem in the areas he needs it most. As self-esteem is built, attitude and behavior will generally improve on their own.

### Building Self-Esteem

Helping a child to have pride in himself is a good start toward building self-esteem. This can be done by making a habit of mentioning any action that is helpful or otherwise positive. At the start, finding things to make mention of may take practice. Many parents are so busy that they rarely take the time to notice the good a child does. Others are simply not used to giving praise. Still others are used to giving only negative feedback.

Remember to commend and compliment a child without patronizing. Don't say to a ten-year-old, "Oh, how beautifully you put your clothes away. It's about time you figured it out." Rather, say, "I appreciate you putting your clothes away. Good job." Although a child may not respond outwardly, he is likely to value what you say and respond positively within himself. This is how self-esteem is built.

There are a number of other things parents and teachers can do to help a child reach and maintain a high level of self-esteem, including those listed here:

#### Instill Confidence
Teaching a child to believe in himself promotes self-confidence and paves the way for attempts at being successful. Once he begins to see positive results from his actions, confidence can continue to grow. It can also help him deal with setbacks and disappointments more easily. Parents and teachers can effectively foster

a child's confidence by setting small goals and issuing appropriate praise when they are reached. As a child gains confidence, he will be likely to develop goals on his own.

### Encourage

Letting a child know that you believe in him can fuel his desire to keep trying. By giving him encouragement, you make it known that you value his efforts and care about his accomplishments.

### Provide Motivation

Giving suggestions on how to accomplish tasks and goals can help motivate a child. Laying the groundwork for activities will increase his chances of success, especially when presented in an interesting or enjoyable way.

### Voice Your Pride

Telling a child that you are proud of him and his accomplishments helps build self-worth, confidence, and determination.

### Teach "Guided" Independence

Children who accomplish tasks and goals on their own experience independence and self-satisfaction. These are important factors in building self-esteem. Providing a child with simple tasks that can be successfully accomplished alone (while under adult supervision) is a good start.

Teaching a child to like himself and become his own best friend can also promote independence, while at the same time giving him the confidence needed to cultivate friendships.

Allowing a child to make choices is another way to help him develop independence. While making choices will present dilemmas and failures along with successes, it can also teach responsibility and help him feel important and worthwhile. Start with small choices, such as deciding on one of two meals for dinner. Keep in mind that since ADHD children often have difficulty making proper choices, they may need assistance in recognizing good decisions.

Each form of independence should be developed gradually and with parental guidance. The level of independence allowed should also be appropriate to age and development. Children should never be left alone without adult supervision as a way of being taught independence.

### Promote Interdependence

Activities that require a child to "do his part" allow interdependence to be experienced. Performing in a skit or playing an instrument in a band are good examples. By encouraging a child to participate in an activity—especially one in which the child has an interest—you help him to become interdependent and value his efforts within a group.

### Be A Good Listener

In order for children to feel valued, they need to be heard and understood. This is especially true of children with ADHD. By carefully listening to what a child has to say, you acknowledge that he is important and help him to develop self-worth.

### Be Supportive

Letting a child know that you are always there for him can make him feel cared for and cared about. This allows him to feel worthwhile, maintain self-esteem, and face disappointment more easily.

### Downplay Small Mistakes

By minimizing the significance of minor incidents, a parent or teacher can lessen discouragement and allow a child to uphold positive feelings about himself.

### Show Appreciation

A parent or teacher can help a child maintain a sense of being valued by thanking him for his efforts on a regular basis.

### Respect Feelings And Emotions

By allowing children to express their feelings and emotions without responding negatively or teasing, you can help them feel respected. In turn, this will help them to maintain self-esteem. Parents and teachers can further show respect for children's feelings and emotions by not placing them in embarrassing situations, and by helping them out of those they get into on their own.

### Have Patience

By being patient (especially under trying circumstances), parents and teachers can help an ADHD child recognize and learn patience. A child who is patient will become less easily frustrated by tasks, and consequently will be less likely to suffer from feelings of inadequacy. Although displaying patience can be quite trying for some adults (especially those with oppositional children), it can help a child to more easily learn skills and maintain or improve self-esteem.

### Rationalize Anger

Parents and teachers often feel resentful of the added time, patience, and effort required by many ADHD children. As a result, they may be quick to display their anger toward an ADHD child. Added life stresses can compound this problem. By giving careful thought to a situation before acting out in frustration, parents and teachers can avoid destroying feelings and lowering self-esteem.

### Show Affection

By giving children hugs or pats on the back, and verbally stating that you love them and you care, you enhance their feelings of being valued and wanted. This is especially important for boys, who often tend to stop receiving affection from their parents as they grow toward adolescence.

### Promote & Support Interests

Providing a child with the physical resources he needs to develop interests can help him build self-esteem and talent. Obtaining a favorite musical instrument and arranging for lessons is a good example.

## Self-Esteem & The Benefits Of ADHD

While most of the focus on having ADHD represents problems and difficulties, there are also positive aspects and benefits. A high percentage of children with ADHD are creative, intelligent, dynamic, interesting, hopeful, kind, and caring. In addition, their impulsivity and constant thought diversion often cause them to notice and appreciate many things others do not. As adults, they frequently become executives in high positions or own their own companies (some studies show that at least 50% of all entrepreneurs have ADHD). Many are solution-oriented and tend to be extremely inventive. Their endless energy, spontaneity, and creativity aid them in being successful and fulfilled.

A number of ADHD children with exceptional qualities encounter problems because their challenges are not well understood. They are, in essence, diamonds in the rough. They need direction and encouragement, especially when they become frustrated.

Most of all, they need self-esteem. Only with these do ADHD children have the tools they need to develop their talents to full potential.

It is important to remember that with high self-esteem even the most unlikely children can make amazing strides. Consider Albert Einstein, who was regarded as stupid and a slow learner by his teachers; Thomas Edison, who was so inattentive his educators thought him to be retarded; and Benjamin Franklin, whose drive and perseverance were the epitome of hyperactivity. These men went on to accomplish great things by turning their difficulties into assets and believing in themselves.

# Chapter Five

## Focal Points
### Improving Attentiveness With Interests & Activities

Helping an ADHD child to improve focus might be likened to channeling an overflow of water from a river. With too much water moving forward, the consequences could be unfavorable; yet stopping the river isn't possible or feasible. Properly routing the water in different directions, however, might be a suitable, and even productive, alternative. This is not to say that a lot of effort won't be required. But the effort invested is likely to prove worthwhile.

Similar to the river having an overabundance of water, an ADHD child may have an excess of distractibility or energy—or both. In this situation, proper direction can also prove to be quite beneficial. And the effort invested in a child can make a vast difference in his life.

### Improving Focus Without Medication

Studies have shown that attentiveness can be improved without medication. In fact, research has suggested that exercise may be just as effective at improving focus as taking stimulant drugs. This may be attributed to the body's release of natural relaxants, known as endorphins, during physical activity.

Other methods of improving focus without medication include self-talk, mental exercises, and the use of memory games. Self-talk, whether done silently to oneself or quietly aloud, can be highly useful in helping a child to stay focused and on task.

Mental exercises in which a child performs a variety of actions in sequence in order to earn an incentive can also be helpful. For example, a parent might tell a child to put away his shoes, let the dog out, and turn off the television (in that order) to earn a small treat. Or the parent might try using the incentive of competition by issuing the same requests and setting a timer to see if the child can complete the tasks before the alarm sounds (this should be done in a playful way that is not threatening or demeaning to the child).

Memory games that require sustained attention are particularly effective for enhancing focus. The game "Simon Says" is a fine example. Played regularly, games that exercise the mind can help a child become conditioned to staying alert.

Children with mild to moderate attentional difficulties tend to make progress at improving focus without medication more quickly than those with severe attentional difficulties. However, even children with extensive problems have shown improvement with the right drug-free therapy.

## The Impact Of Interest

Enjoying the journey through life is important—it is what makes living worthwhile. Liking your profession or the things you do for others can make your life more meaningful and enjoyable. Your interest in what you do can make it easier to stay focused, and help you to maintain structure and consistency in your life. Children are no different. They need interests in order to have goals, gain self-esteem, and build their futures. Children with interests have exciting challenges to conquer, successes to try for, and things to look forward to. As a result, they are less likely to experience depression and more likely to develop friends who share their ideas and enthusiasm.

## Interests And Focus At School

Since school requires a great deal of focusing, ADHD children usually experience most of their focus-related difficulties there. These childrens' tendencies toward being distracted by the slightest diversion can cause them minor difficulty or extreme frustration when it comes to staying on task.

Interests can be extremely useful in helping ADHD children sustain mental focus in school. For example, a child who has an interest in baseball may find school dull and tend to daydream—unless the class studies include some aspect of the sport. Teachers often comment that children "come out of their shells" when the curriculum is related to a subject they enjoy or are curious about.

Since it is not practical for class activities to revolve around an ADHD child's interests, other ways to gain the child's attention must be devised. One teacher recommends taking an "interest inventory" near the beginning of the school year. By finding out what each student's interests are, related assignments can be given out not only to the ADHD child, but also to the other children in class. Interest inventories can easily be updated throughout the year. Utilized properly, this system can be highly effective at promoting children to maintain focus.

In order for any type of interest-based program to be truly successful, assignments must be given in accordance with each child's academic functioning level. Activities that are too difficult can cause frustration and failure rather than the desire to stay focused.

## Other School Considerations

Other practices can also help ADHD children focus better in school. Selecting assignments that are both enjoyable and mildly challenging is a good example. Using incentives is beneficial because it encourages establishing a goal, staying attentive, and reaching completion. Teachers who are inventive and imaginative are likely to come up with a number of helpful ideas. Those who are at a loss for ideas might try what one noted teacher suggests: ask the class.

Allowing a child to help is another effective way to encourage focus while at the same time boosting self-esteem. A fine example of this is peer tutoring, in which a student helps a classmate or younger student with studies. Other forms of helping, such as being a teacher's assistant, are also effective.

## High-Interest Activities

Some activities are interesting enough to keep an ADHD child totally focused. These include watching television, playing computer games, and participating in various high-action sports. The constant movement and instant gratification these activities provide can keep a child's interest for a length of time.

ADHD children often do well with interesting instructional videos and educational computer games. Many parents of ADHD children report an increased interest in learning and better grades at school after setting up an educational computer at home. The fact that some schools are becoming more computer oriented is a plus for ADHD students.

## Effectively Channeling Energies

Sometimes the insight of a parent or teacher can help turn a lack-of-focus problem into a positive situation. For example, a child who spends a great deal of time running around at home or school might be considered a nuisance, while the same child could be seen as talented during track practice. Giving a child the opportunity to "vent" his energies at an acceptable time and place can help him relate to *when* and *where* an activity is appropriate. It can also help him improve attentiveness and develop self-control.

## One-On-One Activities

The consistent interaction one-on-one activities offer is extremely beneficial for most ADHD children. It helps them keep control of their short attention spans and increases their chances of reaching completion.

Some teachers alternate one-on-one activities with group activities when working with ADHD students in the hopes of conditioning better focus. During the one-on-one activities the teacher offers suggestions to a student on how he can remain focused during group activities. If the child shows difficulty during a group activity, the teacher reminds him of the focus techniques taught during the previous one-on-one activity.

At home, one-on-one time may or may not be easier to establish. Parents should try to schedule at least a small amount of time to be spent with an ADHD child every day.

## Interests And Focus At Home

An ADHD child's interests should also be nurtured at home. Children who are actively involved in activities they enjoy are less likely to be a continual source of disturbance to parents and siblings.

Although developing activities related to a child's interests may take some effort on the part of one or both parents, it is time well spent. If possible, involvement in a favorite hobby or sport should be encouraged. Hobbies such as making models or collecting stamps often maintain a child's interest on a daily basis. Best of all, they can be used rain or shine.

Sports can be helpful both in easing hyperactivity and improving attention; however, they need to be carefully chosen. For example, if a child has a sincere desire to play baseball his motivation can help him stay alert during games. On the other hand, a child who selects baseball simply to be involved in a sport might find that waiting his turn at bat requires too much patience, or that being in the outfield offers too many opportunities for distraction.

## Shared Interests

Sharing an interest with an ADHD child can not only help the child improve focus, it can also effectively strengthen the parent-child bond. Finding a common interest is best. That way parents and children can both enjoy the activities (and parents won't be likely to lose focus).

Since it may be difficult dividing time among siblings, and avoiding hard feelings over too much time being spent with one child is likely to be a concern, alternate strategies may need to be used. Some parents share "focus" time spent with an ADHD child between themselves. Others arrange time to be spent with siblings or friends with similar interests.

# Chapter Six

## *School & The ADHD Child*
### Striving For Better Learning Without Medication

School usually presents the most challenge for ADHD children. Here, they are required to sit still and pay attention in order to survive educationally. A high percentage of these children have a need for flexible, adaptive schooling and find that trying to conform is a difficult process. Overcrowded classrooms and high student-to-teacher ratios can contribute substantially to their difficulties. In numerous school systems, the educators and facilities needed to help ADHD children make progress are unavailable. This is mainly due to poor funding and slow implementation of programs.

### Educational Programs

Most schools' academic programs are not designed to accommodate children who have difficulties with hyperactivity and related behaviors. Rather, they are structured according to an educational "plan," and children are expected to adapt. This is a distressing situation for those ADHD children who require different teaching styles and learning atmospheres in order to excel. It can mean the difference between their success or failure. Although some ADHD children can function fairly well in a standard classroom setting, most are unable to perform at their best. In many cases, poor behavior and lack of achievement result, and medication is recommended to make them "fit in."

Ironically, a number of ADHD children who fail behaviorally and academically have high IQs. This further emphasizes the need for adaptive schooling. In effect, school programs and teaching methods need to accommodate the way children learn, rather than medicating children to make them adapt.

## Optimal Learning Environments

Optimal learning environments for ADHD children combine flexibility with behavior management, while teaching social skills and offering remedial help at the same time. Small class sizes are beneficial; they not only lend to increased one-on-one learning, but also tend to be less distracting and can make behavioral management easier. Classes with teachers who are skilled in working with ADHD children and enjoy the challenge of helping them succeed are ideal. In the best of these classes, the teachers are also excellent communicators, and are willing to work closely with parents and their children.

Most ADHD children need as many opportunities as possible to be creative without constant time restraints. They learn best in non-restrictive environments where flexible teaching methods are used. The most effective classes are those in which children do "hands-on" projects for the majority of a school day as opposed to sitting in a chair, reading and writing or listening to lectures. Many parents and professionals feel that not only ADHD children, but all children, could benefit from more flexible teaching styles.

Below are general suggestions from parents and teachers on how to improve the learning environments and educational experiences of ADHD children.

## How Teachers Can Help:

- Make learning fun.
- Give encouragement.
- Teach children to believe in themselves.
- Find the "good" in difficult children and focus on it.
- Be respectful of private issues.
- Avoid speaking negatively about a child to others.
- Be repetitive in a kind manner.
- Get to know your students.
- Help children find their strong points.
- Make your presentations interesting.
- Present lessons in a variety of formats (short lecture, hands-on, cooperative).
- Avoid speaking in a monotone voice.
- Make eye contact when possible.
- Post rules where they are easily visible.
- Remember to have patience.

- Use incentives to promote good behavior.
- Avoid focusing on a child's weaknesses.

## How Parents Can Help:

- Make sure your child has had sufficient sleep.
- Avoid arguments that leave your child in a bad mood when he arrives at class.
- Feed your child a nutritious breakfast.
- Avoid sending your child to school with a lunchbox filled with junk food.
- Make a point of teaching your child neatness and organizational skills.
- Teach your child the "puzzle approach" by showing him how to turn one large task into several smaller tasks.
- Teach your child note writing as a way of remembering things.
- Avoid sending your child to school with toys, shoes that light up, and other distractible items during regular school days.

## Classroom Structure

The way in which a classroom is set up can greatly influence how effectively a child learns. Lighting, temperature, distractions, and seating should all be considered. Large, open classrooms without dividers can be particularly distracting for an ADHD child. Noise can also be a major distraction, therefore

ADHD children should not be seated next to doors, fans, computers, bathrooms, or pencil sharpeners. Window seating is not advisable for most ADHD children. Be sure not to isolate an ADHD child when selecting an appropriate seating arrangement.

Organization within a class is also important; it should not only be practiced by the teacher and aides, but also taught to students. ADHD children benefit from organization in the same way they benefit from routines: they know what to expect.

Nearly all children benefit from an organizing system. Those who have trouble keeping their desks neat are a perfect example. One class with lift-top desks successfully implemented "label graffiti," by making colorful labels for the insides of their desks showing where each item belonged.

## Obtaining The Best Placement

Since most public school programs are not set up to meet the needs of hyperactive and inattentive children, parents often find themselves in frustrating situations. While home schooling or sending a child to a private school may prove to be effective alternatives, these are not options for many families. But there are other things parents can do. First, they can visit their child's school and discuss his needs with a guidance counselor, administrator, school psychologist, or principal, or a combination of these. Then they can inquire if there is a teacher within the child's grade level who is known to work well with hyperactive and inattentive children, and if so, whether the child could attend this teacher's class. Some schools are cooperative in this area, others are not. If your child's school is willing to work with you in this respect, you may be able to utilize the same strategy prior to the beginning of each school year.

A number of parents request special classes for their ADHD children in an attempt to find a more suitable learning setting. One type of special class commonly requested by these parents is a learning disabled or "LD" class. According to many educators, children with ADHD are often placed in LD classes when in fact they should not be. These educators contend that although some ADHD children are behind in their studies, most do not have learning disabilities in the typical sense and may suffer further feelings of inadequacy from this type of placement.

A small percentage of schools currently offer special classes designed specifically for hyperactive and inattentive children. Although some parents and children express dislike over this type of placement, others are pleased with it.

Overall, a special class is what the teacher makes of it. It is less likely that there will be stigma attached to the idea of attending one if it is seen in a positive fashion. Highly motivated teachers can make all the difference. One award-winning teacher successfully turned the image of her special class around so well that children in regular classes wanted to know how they could attend.

Some schools have successfully implemented a behind-the-scenes approach to helping hyperactive and inattentive children. This has been done by intentionally placing them in standard classrooms modeled after optimal learning environments. Here, teachers are familiar with each child's needs and are able to offer sufficient one-on-one attention to students because they have a lower student-to-teacher ratio. There is no stigma. No labeling. Just effective assistance.

## A Teacher's Knowledge of ADHD

Some teachers specialize in ADHD, while others have little or no knowledge of it. A number of teachers don't believe ADHD even exists.

Teachers who are aware of the difficulties associated with ADHD may be easier to communicate with regarding a hyperactive or inattentive child's difficulties and needs. Further, teachers who are familiar with the problems these children face may be more understanding and solution-oriented. For example, one teacher who had researched ADHD noticed that a female student repeatedly asked questions about topics that were already answered in class discussion. After carefully observing this student, the teacher realized that the girl's difficulties were a result of inattention. The teacher helped her student start a simple note-taking system that proved to be very effective (so effective, in fact, that others in the class started using it as well). This teacher's observations, caring, and efforts made a vast difference.

Teachers with no knowledge of ADHD are often eager to learn new ways to help their students. Some parents report extremely good results coordinating with educators who know very little about hyperactivity and inattention. By working together, these parents and teachers effectively help ADHD children toward better educational experiences.

## Communication: The Bridge To Success

Effective ongoing communication between ADHD children, their parents, and their teachers is essential. Only in this way can true educational progress be achieved for these children. Talking with—not at—each other can make a difference for all involved. Take the time to hear what each other has to say. Most importantly, remember to listen to the child's thoughts and concerns.

It is essential not to belittle each other's efforts. More will be accomplished if parents and teachers are open to working together. Those who are tempted to blame a child's problems on each other must come to realize that an ADHD child's problems are not likely to be anyone's fault, and that the real issue at hand is how to find the best possible solutions for the child.

To better understand the differences in a parent-teacher relationship, consider a husband and wife relationship where the husband has a career and the wife stays home managing the house and kids. Each may have a demanding job; however, it might be difficult to visualize the other's hard work. The same can be true of parents' and teachers' efforts. Parents and teachers should keep this in mind when they approach each other.

Teachers should also try to realize that while a child may have numerous difficulties at school, he may have few or none at home. The fact that home is usually less structured than school can be a contributing factor. It may be hard for parents to imagine a child with no difficulties at home having numerous difficulties at school. It is easy to see how this type of situation might lead parents to think the teacher is the problem. To further complicate the situation, a child may cause such class disruption, or require so much attention, that a distressed teacher will approach the child's parents in exasperation and say, "You really need to do something about your child!" As a result, the parents may begin to punish their child for problems encountered during school. This can lead a child to dislike school and his home life—a negative cycle unlikely to accomplish anything positive.

One mother became so flustered by what she felt were inaccurate assessments of her child's behavior at school that she not only asked to visit the class, but also invited the teacher to observe the child at home. After observing the child on each other's "common ground," both were able to see the other's point of view and implement helpful changes.

## Types Of Parent-Teacher Contact

Notes, telephone calls, and conferences are the main forms of communication between a child's parents and teachers. Some teachers prefer only one or two types of contact, while others utilize all three. Because notes may be forgotten or lost, telephone calls and meetings in person are often the preferred forms of communication.

Each type of contact should be used sparingly, unless special circumstances reasonably demand otherwise. Excessive notes and calls from a parent to a teacher (or vice-versa) can be inconvenient and cause harsh feelings to develop.

### Notes

Notes can be used as reminders, thank you's, and mentions of progress or needed improvement. They should not be used repetitively to inform parents of a child's poor behavior. When they are used to report on behavior, they should have an encouraging tone. Rather than writing "Sally's behavior was awful today," a teacher might write "Sally needs to keep trying on her behavior. I know she can do it!" The second approach provides encouragement, preserves a child's self-esteem, and can relieve at least a portion of the child's apprehension in taking the note home (while still getting its point across). The first approach is purely negative, doesn't promote encouragement, and makes the child worry about the consequences she will face at home—the one place many ADHD children find refuge from so many of their challenges.

### Telephone Calls

Telephone contact can be helpful in getting updates on a child's progress, discussing areas of needed improvement, and expressing appreciation, among other things. For many parents and teachers it is the most convenient form of contact. It can be very effective, especially when both parties exercise courtesy by leaving a message or sending a note requesting a return call at a time that is mutually convenient.

Telephone contact should not be used by a teacher to badger a parent about a child's behavior while he or she is at work. Likewise, it should not be used by parents to badger a teacher about a child's lack of progress or other issues while he or she is at work.

### Conferences

Parent-teacher conferences are usually requested periodically throughout the school year. These meetings should be used for making suggestions, finding solutions, and seeing each other's viewpoint. They should not be one-sided or used as a "dumping ground."

Many parents of ADHD children complain that they feel verbally attacked after meetings with their child's teacher. Teachers, on the other hand, often complain that parents do not sufficiently address their children's problems and tend to "lay the load" on teachers.

In order for an ADHD child to make progress in school, quality parent-teacher communication needs to exist. The following charts are comprised of comments from parents and teachers on how to effectively communicate and coordinate with each other during conferences and other times of contact.

## Suggestions From Parents To Teachers:

- Do not approach us angrily about our children's difficulties. Be diplomatic.
- Do not reprimand us as if we were children.
- Try to focus on solutions, not problems.
- Be open to learning about hyperactivity and inattention.
- Give us suggestions, rather than forcing your opinions on us.
- Realize that our children may not have the same problems at home that they face in school.

## Suggestions From Teachers to Parents:

- Express your child's needs at the beginning of the school year.
- Inform your child's teacher of any changes in your child's needs as the year progresses.
- Do not approach teachers angrily about your child's difficulties or lack of progress.
- Be open to suggestions.
- Understand that teachers are required to follow curriculum guidelines.

- Realize that a disruptive child can affect the learning of many other children and that a teacher must alleviate such a situation.
- Avoid arguing with your spouse during a parent-teacher conference.
- Do not expect to meet with your child's teacher every day.
- Make an appointment to meet with your child's teacher, rather than walking in during class instructional time.

## Handling Difficult Situations

Occasionally parents run into problems with a child's teacher. Some teachers are set in their ways and are unwilling to be flexible or accommodating in administering special help to a child. Others disregard parents' concerns and requests, or are particularly hard on a child. Fortunately, these are not common cases.

Although some people recommend approaching the school principal when problems such as these occur, it is important to consider that the child is likely to get caught in the middle between the parents and teacher. In most cases where parents and teachers are unable to come to some form of agreement and maintain reasonable communication, the best alternative is to have the child placed in another class.

The other arena of difficult situations arises when teachers encounter problems with parents. A parent who is unwilling to address a child's difficulties is one example. Sometimes one or both parents are the cause of a child's problems (such as in cases of abuse). In these instances, intervention by school professionals other than the teacher is usually indicated.

## Preserving Self-Esteem At School

As mentioned in chapter 4, self-esteem plays a major role in positive development at school. Here, self-esteem can be affected in many different ways. Most of these involve embarrassment—whether self-inflicted or brought on by the actions of teachers or other students. For example, some teachers reduce children's academic grades as a form of discipline. This not only lowers self-esteem and incites teasing from other students, but also causes an inaccurate indicator of a child's abilities. One teacher who repeatedly disciplined a hyperactive child in this fashion was shocked to find him on her attendance roster for a second year. In addition, the child suffered a considerable loss of self-esteem. It is evident that neither the child nor the teacher benefited from this situation.

Another common form of discipline that can severely affect self-esteem is restricting a child from outdoor physical activities. The embarrassment of not being allowed to participate is often far greater than missing out on the activities themselves. Also, since physical activity has been proven to help lessen hyperactivity and inattention, restricting an ADHD child from participation is obviously counterproductive.

Overall it is best that teachers consider the effects of their actions on children's self-esteem before carrying them out.

## Tutoring

Tutoring can effectively help an ADHD child stay at the same academic level as his peers. There are various types of tutoring, including school-provided tutoring, peer tutoring, parental tutoring, and private tutoring.

School-based remedial tutoring is usually headed by math or reading specialists who are available during or after school hours, or both. These tutors work one-on-one or in small groups with children who require learning assistance. In most schools there is no charge for this service.

Peer tutoring, an effective system in which students assist other students in learning, has become successfully utilized in a number of schools nationwide.

Parental tutoring involves one or both parents working with a child to improve academics. Many parents and children feel parental tutoring brings them closer; however, some find it is too stressful on their relationships. In situations where the latter is the case, private tutoring is often considered. When selecting a private tutor, it is important that parents involve their child in the process. That way they can avoid choosing someone who is not well suited to their child's personality and learning preferences.

## Private Education

For some families, sending an ADHD child to a private school is a viable alternative to public education. When selecting a private school, the academic and social requirements should first be considered, as well as whether the teachers who would be educating your child are knowledgeable in ADHD (or at least flexible and willing to work with your child). As mentioned before, flexibility is beneficial for ADHD children. A private school with high academic demands and strict behavioral guidelines may be more problemsome for an ADHD child than a public school. Some private schools maintain too rigid a structure without flexibility. On the other hand, a private school that offers an individualized educational approach and is willing to help a child improve his social skills may be an excellent alternative to public schooling.

Involving an ADHD child in the process of selecting a private school is important. Forcing a child into a strange new school is not unlike setting him up in a pre-arranged marriage. Although it may work out, making his own selection has many benefits. If the process is more democratic, and the child is allowed to choose from two or more schools, a smooth transition is more likely. Either way, a child may find he likes or dislikes a particular school. Before paying an extended tuition, ask if the child can attend a school day and sit in on classes and activities. Also talk with other parents whose children attend the school, and let your child speak with their children.

## Home Schooling

Another option for some parents of ADHD children is home schooling. This has become an excellent alternative for many parents who have the time, patience, and required skills to teach a child at home. Currently over 20,000 ADHD children are estimated to be home schooled nationwide. Talking with other parents who home school their children, and allowing your child to speak with their children may help you to decide if home schooling would be suitable.

The biggest concern with home schooling has been how a child will develop socially. Surprisingly, many parents have actually reported improved social development in their children. Since home schooling can allow ADHD children to learn at their own pace, away from the scrutiny of other children, they tend to experience less negative interactions with their peers each day. As a result, many of these children gain a new sense of self-esteem and begin to get along better with others.

By involving home-schooled children in supervised extracurricular activities such as sports, parents can help them make new friends and develop socially.

Another concern has been whether home schooling prepares children for the future and "real world" experiences. Parents can help their children in this area by simulating school regimens and by making a point of involving their children in group activities.

When considering home schooling as an option, be sure to check your community's home schooling requirements and find out how to go about registering your child as a home-schooled student.

# Chapter Seven

## *Behavioral Management*
### Making Progress Through Intervention & Guidance

Substantial progress can be made with an ADHD child by using behavioral management. Parents often rely heavily on this type of strategy when medication is ineffective or otherwise cannot be taken by a child. When used properly, behavioral management can increase correct behaviors and decrease or eliminate undesirable ones. A number of different behavioral programs have proven to be useful. Parents should choose a system that is most likely to be effective for their child's particular areas of difficulty, and not be afraid to make changes to it.

It is important to recognize that behavioral management is not restricted to improving inappropriate behaviors such as lying, hitting, or purposefully disrupting class. It can also be useful in helping ADHD children whose behaviors mainly affect themselves, such as those who have difficulty with disorganization, forgetfulness, and daydreaming. Although these behaviors may cause inconvenience for others (such as a parent having to go back to a location to retrieve a forgotten item), the child will be most affected by them in the long run. Since the goal of behavioral management is to implement change, it is often effective in these situations.

## Medication vs. Behavioral Management

Several studies have suggested that there are no long-term behavioral benefits to taking medication for ADHD. In fact, a number of studies have indicated that taking medication as the only form of treatment for ADHD can actually worsen behavior over a period of time. This may be a factor in why some doctors prescribe medication only as a temporary measure until behavioral management has been implemented and a child has shown improvement.

There have been numerous instances in which parents and teachers have successfully helped ADHD children improve their behavioral difficulties without drug therapy. In instances where behavioral management appears to be ineffective, it is usually due to one or more of the following:

- A poorly implemented plan
- Inconsistency
- Attempting to change too many behaviors at once
- A misunderstanding of expectations on the child's part

## Types Of Behavioral Management

The type and level of behavioral management that should be used is as individual as each child. Some children require mild to moderate intervention techniques, while others need more powerful forms of mediation. For example, a child whose difficulties are mainly a problem to himself will not likely need as detailed a behavioral management program as a child who is verbally or physically abusive to others.

Experts have found social skills training, self-instruction, and cognitive-behavioral therapy to be effective forms of behavior management for many children with ADHD. Social skills training teaches a child how to recognize social cues and interact appropriately with others in a variety of situations. This type of skill building is generally taught by a qualified therapist or other professional who discusses various social behaviors, asks and answers questions, and allows a child to "act out" hypothetical social situations. Intensive social skills training should not be reserved for adolescence, but rather should be implemented during the early school years.

Self-instruction, in which a child mentally or verbally reminds himself to perform or avoid certain actions, is an effective form of mental exercise that promotes proper behaviors.

Cognitive-behavioral therapy combines problem-solving and self-instruction skills with behavioral self-monitoring. It can be useful not only in teaching a child how to act and react appropriately in social situations, but also in developing organizational skills and maintaining self-control.

There are many other forms of behavioral management. Some involve the use of incentives and positive reinforcement, while others are based solely on issuing negative consequences. For most ADHD children, a flexible combination of these types of management is most effective. The best systems appear to be those in which incentives are many and negative consequences are mild.

No matter what type of behavioral management is implemented, infractions should be considered individually in conjunction with a child's difficulties. For example, an inattentive child who forgets to bring his book to school should not be punished, rather he should be assisted in remembering through the use of reminder labels or incentives.

## Behavioral Management At School

In order for behavioral management to be successful, it needs to be implemented at school as well as at home. Unfortunately, an effective behavioral system used by parents at home may not be the same system used by their child's teacher. This may cause some confusion for the child, who finds it necessary to "shift gears" from a classroom-oriented behavioral system to a home-based system after school. Since a teacher's behavior-management techniques are usually designed for class situations which involve numerous children, it is unlikely that he or she will be willing to modify the program for one child. In addition, while some teachers are flexible in their behavioral approaches with individual children, others do not appreciate being told how to discipline or assist a child. Making an effort to see each other's point of view may help parents and teachers work better together toward developing a system that is effective both at home and at school. Some parents find it helpful to observe the behavioral system a teacher uses during class in order to devise a similar program to use at home.

## The Importance Of Consistency

Implementing and maintaining a behavioral program takes time, patience, and tireless effort. Parents, children, and teachers must continually remain actively involved. A behavioral program that is not constantly followed is unlikely to yield positive results.

Consistency among parents is one of the most important factors in establishing an effective behavioral regime. A lack of it is the main reason most behavioral management programs fail. Parents who discuss and set rules, and decide upon suitable forms of discipline and assistance *before* a program is implemented often report the best results. Those who persistently maintain a program are likely to see long-term effects from their efforts.

## Seeking Professional Assistance

When behavior management attempted by parents and teachers proves ineffective, the services of a behavioral specialist may be useful. These therapists specialize in developing and implementing programs that address specific areas of behavior-related difficulty. Their services often prove beneficial when:

- Parents are unable to come to a suitable agreement on how to manage their child's difficulties
- Parents are overwrought with problems or responsibilities and have difficulty successfully implementing behavior-management techniques
- Parents have opposing parenting styles
- Parents are divorced and require outside mediation
- Parents are in continual conflict
- Teachers request additional assistance in implementing a behavioral program
- Children are unresponsive to behavioral strategies

## Counseling & Psychotherapy

Various forms of individual and family counseling and psychotherapy have proven helpful to a number of ADHD children and their families. Individual counseling is useful in dealing with the specific needs and concerns of each family member. Family counseling allows all members to air issues and work toward solutions with the aid of a therapist, psychologist, or psychiatrist. Working towards solutions enables family members to discover and develop the family's resources and strengths. It also helps parents regain deteriorating patience and motivation.

Psychotherapy appears to be most useful with ADHD children who are anxious, depressed, angry, or withdrawn, or have a severe lack of self-esteem.

Counseling in any form is an invasive process. For those who do not care to share their problems with others it can be an uncomfortable one. It is therefore essential that the professional selected to work with a child and his family is not only qualified, but also caring, respectful, and solution-oriented.

## Parent Training

Since raising a child is not an inborn trait, and raising an ADHD child can be particularly challenging, parents sometimes need assistance and direction. Researching the successful methods used by others may be beneficial. This can be done by asking the parents of other children what has and has not worked for them, and why. Also consider taking a parenting course.

One mother who initially described her daughter as "unable to control herself" without medication found both a behavior management program *and* a parenting program to be helpful. Her daughter was on Ritalin for seven years, and neither she nor her husband had previously considered trying a behavioral program. Within six months after starting one, their daughter was able to function well without medication and had mastered several social skills. In addition, both parents had enrolled in a parenting program where they learned a number of effective parenting techniques. Most importantly, they gained insight into the impact of making negative comments to their daughter and others regarding her difficulties. They also learned the importance of giving her praise and encouragement on a regular basis.

Although most ADHD children's difficulties are not caused by poor parenting, many parents can benefit from a parenting program.

# Chapter Eight

## Diet & Nutrition vs. Drug Therapy
### Food For Thought

There has been considerable debate over whether certain foods and additives cause hyperactivity and related behaviors. According to some reports, only 5% of hyperactive and inattentive children experience diet-induced ADHD symptoms. Several studies and surveys, however, have indicated a much higher percentage, and suggest that these symptoms can be improved, controlled, or eliminated through proper nutrition and simple changes in diet.

Opting for dietary control of symptoms over drug therapy eliminates the risk of medication-induced side effects. In addition, research has shown that it can greatly improve a child's overall health. Many parents use dietary methods of controlling hyperactivity and inattention when drug therapy is contraindicated.

### The Feingold Theory & Program

Much of the focus on diet and how it affects children's behavior began in 1975 when a pediatrician and allergist by the name of Benjamin Feingold published a book titled *Why Your Child Is Hyperactive*.

In it, Feingold cited synthetic food dyes, chemical preservatives, foods containing salicylates, and artificially manufactured flavorings as the causes of hyperactivity in numerous children.

Not long after the publication of his book, "Feingold groups" appeared across the country. These groups were made up of parents who shared menu ideas and recipes, and devised tactics to keep children away from the behavior-altering foods.

Within months, dramatic behavioral changes were reported by thousands of parents who implemented Feingold's program. Yet despite the apparent validity of his findings, skeptics contended that the behavioral improvements in these children were attributed to the extra attention they were afforded while their diets were being modified, and not to the program itself. Defenders of the program disputed such an idea, stating that if this was true, parents' attempts at other forms of intervention would have yielded the same results. The arguments of other opposers were often just as unfounded, and mainly due to misinformation.

Most of the criticism aimed at the Feingold program over the years has come from food chemical manufacturers and others in the food trade. Their reactions only make sense, considering that the vast majority of foods available in stores contain synthetic additives, and widespread avoidance by consumers could have a severe financial impact on the industry.

A number of studies sponsored by the food industry to validate the effectiveness of the Feingold diet were reportedly plagued with discrepancies and yielded inconclusive or inaccurate results. Nevertheless, the food industry published numerous materials denouncing the program and distributed them publicly.

In spite of the food industry's negative stance, a multitude of children continue to benefit from the Feingold program today. Parents consistently report that it is an effective method of symptom control for ADHD. Further, research has shown over a 50% success rate when the program is properly followed.

## Time Investment, Cost, & Restrictions

Although some parents believe that using the Feingold program would be costly and overly time-consuming, the opposite is usually true. The majority of parents report spending less on grocery costs. The time invested in reading labels is minimal because the program includes lists of foods to avoid.

Contrary to the beliefs of some opposers, the Feingold program *does not* eliminate sweets and *does* include a variety of allowable snack foods. Several of the restricted foods and food additives are discussed below, along with a look at the effects of artificial sweeteners, caffeine, and sugar.

### *Synthetic Colors*
Synthetic food dyes derived from coal tar or petroleum are used in a number of foods including cookies, crackers, fruit drinks, lunch meats, cheeses, ice cream,

and numerous other packaged goods. Although the FDA certifies several synthetic colors for use in foods, many are inadequately tested.

A number of studies have shown that artificial color additives increase hyperactivity and other related problems in children. One study included 200 children who were given a diet free of synthetic coloring for six weeks. The parents of 150 of these children noted improved behaviors with the removal of the synthetic colors from the childrens' diets, and deteriorating behaviors when the colors were reintroduced.

### Preservatives

Similar to synthetic colors, artificial preservatives may cause chemical reactions in the brain that disturb the production of neurotransmitters and cause hyperactivity, inattention, and other behavioral changes. Those most commonly used are:

- **BHA** (butylated hydroxyanisole)—an antioxidant often found in cereals, baked goods, meat products, and snack foods.

- **BHT** (butylated hydroxytoluene)—an antioxidant often used along with BHA in cereals, baked goods, meat products, and other packaged foods.

- **TBHQ** (tertiary butylhydroquinone)—an antioxidant frequently used in conjunction with BHT and BHT.

- **Sulfites** (ammonium sulfite, sodium sulfite, sodium bisulfite, sodium metabisulfite, potassium bisulfite, potassium metabisulfite, and sulfur dioxide)—sulfur-based antioxidants used in wine, seafood, dried fruits, jellies, vinegars, salad dressings, cookies, and other foods. Also used as bleaching agents.

- **Nitrites and Nitrates**—Preservatives used for the prevention of botulism in ham (both packaged and canned), lunch meat, hot dogs, sausage, bacon (including dried bacon pieces used in salads), pork, and other meat products.

Each of these preservatives carries additional health risks and should be avoided. Nitrites in particular have been linked to brain damage.

### Artificial Flavorings

There are literally hundreds of chemicals used to replace natural flavors. Many produce hyperactivity in children; however it is often impossible to track down which ones are the offenders since most of them are lumped under the title "artificial flavoring" on ingredient panels. For many children, avoidance of all artificial flavorings is best.

### Flavor Enhancers

Flavor enhancers are additives used to draw out or accentuate the flavors of foods and other additives. Monosodium glutamate, also known as MSG, is the most commonly used flavor enhancer.

Past research on MSG showed destruction of nerve cells in the brains of infant mice who were fed large amounts of the additive. Soon after, baby food companies eliminated MSG from their products (possibly as a result of consumer pressure).

MSG is used in foods from soup to nuts, literally. Although it is often listed on food labels as "monosodium glutamate," it may also be a component of other food ingredients such as "yeast extract" or "hydrolyzed vegetable protein."

Parents whose children experience "Chinese restaurant syndrome" (burning, tingling, or pressure in the upper body and/or headache and nausea) or other sensitivities after consuming MSG should carefully check ingredient panels. Although numerous studies had previously been unable to find a link between MSG and these side effects, recent research by the Food and Drug Administration confirmed that the additive adversely affects various people.

Another flavor enhancer which has come under scrutiny for possible brain chemistry alteration and adverse behavioral effects is the artificial sweetener aspartame. Although its general use is in sweetening cereals, baked goods, drinks, pills and vitamins (especially chewables), dessert mixes, and yogurt, it is also used to enhance the sweetness of sucrose (table sugar) in a number of baked goods, candies, and gum.

## Salicylates

Salicylates are natural compounds. They are used in aspirin and are found in the following foods, beverages and spices:

- almonds
- apples & apple cider
- apricots
- berries
- cherries
- chili powder
- cider vinegar
- cloves
- coffee
- cucumbers
- currants
- grapes
- mint
- nectarines
- oranges
- peaches
- bell peppers
- chili peppers
- pickles
- plums
- prunes
- raisins
- tangerines
- tea
- tomatoes
- wine

Salicylates are believed to cause behavioral problems in some children by disturbing the brain's ability to produce neurotransmitters. Interestingly, a child may be sensitive to one salicylate-containing food, while showing no signs of sensitivity to another. The Feingold diet recommends temporarily eliminating these items from the diet and then adding them back one at a time to confirm any changes in behavior.

## Artificial Sweeteners

Saccharin and aspartame are presently the most commonly used artificial sweetening agents; however, the safety of both has been questioned. Saccharin is between 250 and 750 times sweeter than sucrose and is used in a variety of products including gum, candy, soft drinks, and dessert mixes. Although it has been on the market for over 70 years, in more recent years tests have shown the sweetener causes bladder cancer. As a result, all products containing saccharin are now required to carry cancer warnings.

Aspartame, known to consumers under the brand name Nutrasweet, is approximately 200 times sweeter than sucrose. It was introduced into the food market in July of 1981 after the FDA approved its use for all but those with phenylketonuria (PKU).

Many scientists and doctors believe aspartame may be a cause of behavioral problems in children. In his book *Environmental Poisons in Our Food*, Dr. J. Gordon Millichap states that aspartame blocks the normal increases in brain serotonin produced by a carbohydrate meal. Serotonin is one of the main neurotransmitter chemicals in the brain responsible for controlling hyperactivity. The less serotonin there is in the blood, the more hyperactive a child is likely to become.

In 1984 the Center for Disease Control (CDC) investigated reports of behavioral and neurological disturbances including headaches and mood changes after the consumption of aspartame. In response, the CDC acknowledged that some persons may be particularly sensitive to the sweetener.

## Caffeine

Caffeine is a natural stimulant found in tea, coffee, sodas (including non-cola types), cocoa, and chocolate. It can cause anxiety, nervousness, behavioral changes, and stimulation of the central nervous system; however, these symptoms are usually temporary.

Due to its stimulant properties, caffeine has been used as a treatment for ADHD. While some studies indicate that its use may increase the production of neurotransmitters in the brain, the dosage requirements would likely be high and thus outweigh the benefits in terms of side effects.

## Sugar

Refined sugar has long been a suspect in children's overactivity (with the average American child eating 150 pounds of sugar annually, it is easy to see why). Yet while many parents comment that their children display hyperactive or moody behavior after consuming sugar-containing foods, controlled studies have not proven such an effect. Only a small percentage of children have been shown to be sensitive to sugar, usually in the form of an allergy.

Considering that most sugar-based junk foods contain synthetic dyes and other additives, it may be that these ingredients eaten in conjunction with sugar are the offending substances, rather than the sugar itself.

Nevertheless, sugar does not contribute sound nutrients to any diet and has been linked to a number of physical disorders including diabetes and hypo-glycemia. Hypoglycemia can affect concentration and mood throughout each day, and symptom control depends heavily on quality nutrition.

## Nutrition And Brain Function

Nutrition is essential for proper brain function. Correct eating habits not only provide the body with the nutrients necessary to grow, but also enhance thought processes. Two chemical compounds within the body, glucose and glutamic acid, are used to regulate brain activity. Both are derived from foods.

Low levels of chromium in the blood can affect glucose metabolism, as well as the utilization of protein. Numerous children are deficient in chromium as a result of poor diet habits and excess consumption of junk foods.

Protein is essential because it produces the amino acid tyrosine. A deficiency of tyrosine in the diet inhibits the production of norepinephrine, another main neurotransmitter in the brain. High-protein foods include beans, cheese, nuts, seeds, yogurt, fish, meat, and turkey.

## Vitamins And Supplements

Some studies have indicated that food additives may actually decrease the body's ability to utilize nutrients, with hyperactivity as a result. The inhibited metabolization of vitamin B6 (pyroxidine) due to the consumption of artificial additives is of particular concern because it is utilized in a greater number of physical and mental body functions than any other nutrient and is essential for normal brain and nervous system function.

Vitamins and supplements filled with synthetic additives may actually defeat their own purpose. It is usually best to select natural vitamins from a health food store.

## In Conclusion

All factors considered, it is evident that a well-balanced diet which is high in protein, low in sugar, and free of synthetic colorings, preservatives, and additives can be useful in enhancing concentration and attention in children and improving overall health.

# Chapter Nine

## *From A Child's View*
### Children's Feelings About ADHD & Drug Therapy

Children who are diagnosed with ADHD have distinct thoughts and concerns. Their views about having a disorder can cause them to feel confused, upset, and overwhelmed. Being required to take medication for their difficulties can intensify these feelings.

Although some ADHD children experience an initial sense of relief after learning their problems have a cause, negative feelings often catch up with them in the long run. A number of children become depressed when told that their challenges may be permanent, or that there is the possibility they will need to take medication for the rest of their lives. Others wonder how ADHD and drug therapy will affect their bodies, their careers, their relationships, and their futures.

Unfortunately, children's views and concerns are often overlooked during the development of treatment plans. Yet these are the areas that require the most attention from parents, teachers, and doctors in order to effectively help hyperactive and inattentive children toward improvement.

Numerous professionals feel that the biggest challenges for ADHD children lie in developing self-esteem and improving relationships with their peers. For many children, a diagnosis of ADHD is more debilitating to self-esteem than being undiagnosed and struggling with difficulties. And while in some instances peer relationships improve when a child begins drug therapy, in many others they deteriorate further. This commonly happens when other children are alerted to the idea that an ADHD child has a "problem" and needs to take medication.

With these factors in mind, parents and doctors need to seriously consider the impact of telling a child he has ADHD. In addition, they must try to perceive the initial and long-term emotional effects of placing a child on drug therapy.

The remainder of this chapter provides insight into how children feel about ADHD in general, as well as their reactions to being diagnosed with the condition and their views on drug therapy.

## How Children View ADHD

Most children don't know anything about ADHD. Additionally, many are confused about it even after they have been given an explanation. Those who have a brother, sister, classmate, or teammate with ADHD sometimes have a clearer perception of it; however, this is not always the case. Here are comments from non-ADHD children when asked "What do you think Attention Deficit Hyperactivity Disorder is?":

"I don't know, but it doesn't sound good."

"I'm not sure. Is it contagious?"

"I think it's a sickness or something that makes you mean and makes you talk a lot. A kid on my baseball team has it."

"I think it's when you're born with a brain that doesn't think right. My sister's got it. It makes her a real pain. She's always sloppy and interrupts people and forgets things."

"I'm pretty sure it's a sickness that makes people mental. That's what my best friend told me."

"I think it's what they call it when you're hyper and you feel like running around."

"I' m not really sure. My parents said my brother has it, though. They say he just has trouble sitting still and being quiet because his mind thinks slow, but I think they're lying. I think it's something in your brain that can make you die."

"Who knows? Not me. Do you think I have it?"

"I think it's something that makes you sick and makes you act bad at school."

"It's a problem with your brain that never gets better. My brother's got it."

It is evident that there is some misconception about ADHD among children who don't have it. But in many instances, they are not the only ones who are confused. When asked to describe ADHD, the comments from children who have been diagnosed with it are often just as distressing. Here are just a few:

"It's a problem with your brain nobody can fix."

"It's when you have too many chemicals in your head and they make you jumpy."

"I can't describe it too good. I don't think my mom can either. It's what they say you have when you have a lot of problems in school."

"It's like a sickness in your brain that makes you think fast and act fast. I still haven't figured out what the big deal about it is."

"It's what doctors call it when you have trouble sitting still and paying attention."

"All I can tell you is it's a problem with your mind that makes it hard to think and sit still."

"I'd say it's when your brain tells your body to do things too fast."

"You're born with it. Your brain doesn't work right."

"It's a brain disease you catch from your parents."

"It's a sickness."

*Additional Insight*

Most parents whose children have been told they have ADHD are shocked to hear their sons and daughters describe what ADHD is. Often the thoughts parents tried to convey to their child about ADHD are not the same as those the child actually has. One study showed that nearly 90% of ADHD children have a different perception of ADHD than what was described by their parents and doctors.

## How ADHD Children React To The Diagnosis

Most children who are told they have ADHD struggle with a mixture of emotions. Many are worried, ashamed, or angry, and wonder "Why me?" Some blame themselves or their parents for their "problem." Others become jealous of children who do not have the same difficulties.

Since describing ADHD usually involves some mention of how a person thinks or how his brain functions, a number of children who are told they have it become overwrought with concern and believe there is something seriously wrong with them. Some children actually think they will die from ADHD. This is not as outlandish as one might think, especially considering the fact that emotional overarousal is a symptom of ADHD. It does, however, promote some consideration for thought on how to approach a child about his difficulties.

Older ADHD children and those with high intelligence levels may attempt to do some "research" on the diagnosis on their own. What they uncover may be confusing and frighten them. This is another reason why labeling may best be avoided.

## How ADHD Children Feel About The Diagnosis

Beyond their views on what ADHD is and how they feel about having it, many older ADHD children have opinions about whether they should have been told they have a disorder, or whether their difficulties should have been addressed without being labeled. The following quotes are from children ages 14 to 17 who were asked the question, "Has it helped you to know you have ADHD, or would you rather have not known and simply had someone help you learn how to pay attention and use your energies in better ways?"

"It's hurt me more than helped me. I would have rather had someone help me with my problems without making me feel like a reject."

"It definitely hasn't helped me. For the past three years since they told me and my teachers I have it, I've been left out of more class activities than I can count."

"It helped me in the beginning because my teachers seemed to understand why I had so much energy. Now I'm back to where I started. Only now they always ask me if I've taken my medicine. It makes you feel low, you know?"

"Of course it hasn't helped me. People only think bad things about kids with ADD. When you get to be a teenager it gets worse. Everyone seems to see you as a problem with a problem. I don't like knowing, but mostly I don't like other people knowing and it seems like everyone does."

"At this point it doesn't matter either way."

"I don't think I should have been told, but I never believed it anyway. The worst part is when your teachers and counselors want to talk to you about it. They have no idea how you feel and most of them really don't want to help you."

## Additional Insight

A child whose concerns are adequately addressed without labeling is likely to make progress. Further, a child whose views are reflected in his improvement program is apt to show more interest and a greater desire to participate. For example, a child who is behind academically may say he is embarrassed because he can't read at the same level as his peers. An improvement plan that includes tutoring in reading could effectively address this child's concerns. The idea that such a system will help him read better and lessen his embarrassment can make him want to participate.

## How ADHD Children Feel About *Not* Being Labeled

For a percentage of ADHD children the issue is not what they think of having been labeled, but rather why they weren't. Some wish they had been, and others are glad they never were. Here are varied views from hyperactive and inattentive children between 13 and 17 years of age who were asked how they would feel now if they knew their difficulties were related to a disorder:

"I guess I'd be glad there was a reason for my problems. But I'm not really sure. I never thought about it before."

"I wouldn't care. I'd laugh. I don't have a disorder. I just have a lot of energy and I use it."

"I'd think it would have been nice to know sooner so I would have understood things better. But I guess it might have caused me more problems with other kids and stuff."

"I'd be glad my parents never told me. I wouldn't have liked being treated like a geek by everybody."

"I think I'd be confused."

"I'd be totally glad my parents didn't make a fool out of me."

### Additional Insight

Labeling is not necessary to help a child toward improvement. Many hyperactive and inattentive children who are not labeled ADHD improve to a greater extent than those who are.

## How Children See Drug Therapy

Children learn the following equation early on:

$$Medication = Sick$$

As a result, no matter what a child is told about drug therapy, he will be likely to develop his own inner stigma about the need to take medication.

Some parents and doctors compare taking medication to wearing eyeglasses when explaining drug therapy to a child. But likening medication to eyeglasses still emphasizes that there is a problem that needs correction, rather than skills that need direction. Only from a child's view, there is a big difference. Their "problem" isn't with their eyes. It is with their mind.

Another reason why the eyeglasses analogy is inappropriate is that while many eye problems are permanent, the symptoms of ADHD may not be. According to several studies, many children "outgrow" ADHD. Most of this research indicates vast improvement in symptoms during adolescence. Whether the symptoms improve due to physiological changes in the body during puberty, or increased effort in compensating for difficulties due to peer pressure, the fact remains that a number of ADHD children—as many as 50% or more according to some studies—*do* improve.

Below are general comments about drug therapy from ADHD children:

"It really makes me angry when kids tease me about my medicine during Say No To Drugs week."

"I'll never be able to get a job because they'll know I take drugs."

"My parents said my brain does what it wants to so I need to take medicine to control it. I really don't like it though."

"I know my future's shot. I'll never get the job I want because when they do a drug test they'll know I take Ritalin."

"I get teased a lot because I take medicine to slow me down."

"I know my medicine helps me, but I'd rather not take it because it makes me feel sick."

"A lot of adults treat you strange when they know you take medicine for being hyper. I don't like that."

"I really feel like I need the medicine, but I wish there was another way because it's embarrassing always needing to take it."

"I don't like having to take medicine when I don't feel like I need it."

"My brother teases me about taking my medicine and my sister feels sorry for me. I just can't stand it anymore."

### Additional Insight

A number of ADHD children become frustrated over being required to take medication when they feel they can do well without it. Others feel it is helpful sometimes, but not always, and would rather take it occasionally. Some feel they are forced to take it.

Other concerns ADHD children have about drug therapy include embarrassment over a teacher or school nurse giving medication, and comments from other children about taking "crazy pills," "chill pills," or "spaz drugs."

## Imperfect Perfection

The fact that our society is geared toward perfection makes dealing with ADHD even harder on children. Not only do most children want to fit in with their peers and be seen as "normal" by parents, teachers, friends, and relatives, they also want to accomplish goals, feel pride, and in one way or another be considered "perfect." In the eyes of many children, being labeled as having a disorder and placed on drug therapy eliminates that opportunity.

# Chapter Ten

## *All In The Family*
### Making Drug-Free Therapy Work At Home

A child's difficulties due to hyperactivity and inattention usually affect his entire family. The inconveniences and annoyances to parents and siblings can range from being minor to being so severe that daily home life becomes a continuous, frustrating struggle. When the latter is the case, family members (especially parents) often become physically and emotionally drained.

While medicating a child for ADHD might allow family interactions and stresses to improve, it carries with it the many drawbacks and contraindications discussed throughout this book. Drug-free therapy, on the other hand, frequently proves to be just as effective—if not more so—when utilized properly.

This chapter focuses on improving family life with an ADHD child by making drug-free therapy work at home. It includes proven suggestions and helpful insight from parents and siblings of hyperactive and inattentive children.

## The Family As A Team

Improving home life with an ADHD child takes understanding, effort, and cooperation. Parents need to see eye-to-eye on a number of issues in order for effective change to take place. Together they must help the child meet his needs, while at the same time teaching him how to recognize and apply appropriate behaviors. Further, parents must alert siblings to various ways they can help in the improvement process.

A team effort is essential not only in implementing good family relations but also in maintaining them. Communication between family members must be ongoing, and problems must be addressed and resolved as they arise. In addition, parents and siblings must make a habit of working toward solutions, rather than placing blame and arguing.

In cases where parents are in extreme conflict and feel they cannot effectively help their child, or siblings have high levels of anger and resentment toward an ADHD child, therapy may be helpful. Through therapy many families are able to resolve problems that would otherwise interfere with their attempts to improve home life.

## Parental Attitude About ADHD

Each parent's attitude about ADHD can have a bearing on family life, as well as on interactions with a hyperactive or inattentive child. Some parents see

ADHD as a valid condition, others don't. Either way, it is important that parents are willing to acknowledge that their child has difficulties, if in fact he does. Parents who refuse to acknowledge a child's challenges cannot successfully promote improvement. Those who show understanding and support, however, often see major changes. As one father commented, "I wasn't about to label my daughter disordered. But letting her know that I understood she had some struggles to overcome made a real difference for our whole family."

On the other hand, parents who constantly refer to their son or daughter as having ADHD (and make a point of telling everyone) also do their child a great disservice. A mother of two who felt she learned this the hard way remarked, "I guess that by telling everyone my son had ADHD I was trying to let myself off the hook about being seen as a bad parent. I didn't realize how it was affecting him until I found him crying in his room one afternoon and he told me. I never felt worse in my life. It's just not worth it to label your child ADHD."

## Parents' Feelings

### Grief

Many parents go through a grieving process after being told their child has ADHD. This is frequently attributed to the way ADHD is described to parents. All too often doctors present the diagnosis as a disorder that needs to be controlled with medication.

Rarely do they mention the benefits, or how to bring about improvement without drug therapy.

Viewing a child's difficulties as a challenge rather than a burden can make a substantial difference in family life as well as in a parent's outlook and feelings. Seeing an ADHD child as energetic, impulsive, and in need of direction can be much more productive than seeing him as a child with a disorder which causes him to be problemsome. As one mother said: "When my doctor told me that my youngest son had ADHD, and explained that is was a form of brain dysfunction, I went into shock. At first I felt guilty and depressed. It was horrible. The more I read about ADHD the worse I felt. Out of guilt I started spending more time with him. That was the best thing I could have done. It made me realize that he had many special talents that simply needed direction. Now I focus on the pluses of ADHD and teach my son how to use his energies productively."

*Resentment*

In addition to other emotions, parents often feel resentful over having to devote so much time and effort into helping an ADHD child. This resentment can also cause guilt. To overcome such feelings, parents need to make time for themselves whenever possible. This is evident in the following comments from the mother of a seven-year-old girl: "It was getting to the point where if my daughter even asked me to pass the salt I wanted to scream at her. It seemed like she was invading my every moment. She was constantly talking and always busy. Then one of my friends pointed out that I was spending too much time with my daughter and none by myself. She also suggested that I find an interest for my daughter. So I went out shopping alone and bought my daughter a bead kit to keep her busy. What a difference! Now I go out alone at least once a week and I make a point of finding new projects for her to do."

### Frustration

Parents of ADHD children often experience frustration. Despite their many attempts to help their children improve, it sometimes seems as though nothing works. It is important for parents to maintain hopeful attitudes and keep trying. In most cases it is simply a matter of finding the right system for a particular child. As the mother of one ADHD teenager stated, "By the time my son was eleven I was ready to lose my mind. I tried everything I could possibly think of short of medicating him to help him control his hyperactivity and inattention at school. The teachers just didn't want to deal with him. Then a school counselor suggested testing him to find out what type of atmosphere he learned best in. After testing my son she recommended he be placed in classes with "least restrictive atmospheres." The class changes she made for him literally changed his life and mine too. Now it's a pleasure to talk with his teachers. There's a lot less stress. Best of all, my son actually looks forward to going to school."

## Parental Self-Esteem

Parents—especially mothers—of ADHD children often develop low self-esteem. Constant criticism of their parenting techniques and the actions of their children are usually the main causes.

It is important for parents of ADHD children to maintain good self-esteem and a positive outlook. Only in this way can they effectively help their children toward improvement. As one mother said, "I came to realize that my efforts were worthwhile in spite of unproductive criticism. Rather than dwelling on what others thought of me, I focused my efforts on helping my daughter manage her hyperactivity. Being proud of her progress helped both of us feel better about ourselves."

## Taking Care Of Yourself And Your Spouse

Tending to the needs of any family is a time-consuming challenge. But the added requirements of managing a family with an ADHD child can cause parents to feel additional fatigue both physically and emotionally. It is therefore important that such parents get sufficient rest and take time for relaxation away from their children.

Parents should try to arrange at least two getaways alone each year, even if they are short ones. Evenings alone should be arranged weekly if possible. Although those with several children and tight budgets may find little time and money for themselves, they need to realize that they are usually most in need of time alone. Mothers who tend to ADHD children all day every day should be relieved of caring for them once a week at minimum. This is especially important for mothers who home school. If this is not possible, mothers should try to spend quiet time for themselves while their children sleep.

## ADHD Parent/ADHD Child

Parents sometimes say they see their children struggling with many of the same difficulties they did as children. As these adults read about ADHD, they often say they see themselves in the description. If in fact ADHD can be inherited (which scientific studies have yet to prove), parents should not feel guilty for passing the traits to their children. Rather than concentrating on the negative, these parents should feel fortunate that they can better relate to what their children are feeling. Together they can make many strides toward improvement.

## Two ADHD Children

One mother began seeing many of the same ADHD characteristics in her youngest son that were evident in her older son. Rather than becoming depressed that her younger child was also having difficulties, she expressed that the experience and confidence she gained working with her older son would help her to effectively develop her younger son's talents and minimize his difficulties. This mother's positive attitude helped both of her children make progress.

## Sibling Rivalry And ADHD

Problems among siblings may be more frequent when one or more children in the same family have ADHD. Part of this can be attributed to a non-ADHD child's frustration over an ADHD brother or sister's aggressiveness, messiness, moodiness, or other annoying characteristics. Non-ADHD siblings may also feel left out or neglected if their parents spend an excess of time with the ADHD child. This can cause them to act resentful toward a brother or sister.

Sibling rivalry situations that involve ADHD children often arise out of misunderstandings. Because many ADHD children tend to think accidents are intentional, their impulsive responses may cause them to strike a sibling who has inadvertently bumped into them. Social skills training can be extremely useful in teaching these children how to recognize and acknowledge accidental actions.

## Taking Care Of Siblings

When an ADHD child requires considerable time and effort on the part of one or both parents, siblings may feel that the child is the favorite, or may see him as a problem. These feelings can be alleviated to some extent by allowing siblings to help the ADHD child with easy tasks. It is important, however, that parents take care not to overburden siblings with the ADHD child's needs. Most importantly, parents need to spend time with their non-ADHD children in order to make them feel cared for and worthwhile.

## Devising Routines That Work

ADHD children usually do best when they know what to expect. As a result, regular routines and schedules can be very helpful to them. Here are some tips from parents of ADHD children on how to make daily routines run more smoothly:

### Morning
- Find out which system works best for waking your child: you or an alarm clock.
- Let your child make a recording telling himself what he needs to do each morning. Play the recording as soon as he wakes up each day.
- Post a list of things to be done each day in the child's bedroom. Make morning, afternoon, and evening categories.
- Set a timer that shows the child how long he has to get ready for school.
- If your child wakes up in a bad mood, don't add to it. Be positive and encouraging. Try to find out what's troubling the child. In many instances,

ADHD children are just frustrated by the prospect of facing another day of school. Give suggestions and encouragement.

- Provide your child with a nutritious breakfast. Give two or more food options when possible.
- Allow enough time for all morning tasks to be completed without rushing.
- If possible, take your child to school.

*After School*
- If your child attends after-school care, be sure to explain his areas of difficulty to the director of the program, and provide recommendations on what to do if problems arise.
- If your child comes directly home from school each day, write a short list of easy things for him to do when he arrives. Have him cross off each item as he completes it and then report to you for snack time, free time, or other activities.
- Take the time to assist your child with homework or look over his schoolwork for the day.

*Evening*
- Have your child select his clothing for the next school day.
- Direct your child in the preparation of his lunch for the next school day.
- Make sure your child places homework or other school papers in his backpack or folder, or an area where they won't be forgotten.
- Allow your child to help with dinner preparation or table setting.

*Bedtime*
- Make sure your child brushes his teeth, straightens his room, or completes other required tasks before being tucked in or read to.
- Leave at least one half hour each night for "tuck-in time." This includes reading stories, giving back massages, etc. If you have several children, you may need to adjust this amount of time.
- If you have more than one child, consider reading bedtime stories as a group.

*Weekends*
- Attempt to stay consistent with the regular weekly routine for waking up.
- Arrange activities that your child can do during the weekend prior to the weekend's arrival. That way you can make sure you have any necessary supplies. If your child is a teenager, have him write a list of activities he would like to do and then discuss them with him.
- Do individual activities as well as family activities with your children.

*General Suggestions*
- Find a babysitter who is patient and responsible. Explain any special concerns up front.
- Avoid taking a child out in pubic unless he can display appropriate behavior. Use incentives.
- Teach your child to recognize inappropriate actions and why it is important to avoid them.

- Provide your child with a brightly colored tape dispenser to be used to tape homework or school notes to an area near the front door.
- Select comfortable clothing for your child.
- Set consequences for disturbing others' belongings and stick to them.
- Help direct your child in cleaning his room, either verbally or with a list. It can be difficult for a distractible child to clean and organize alone.
- Ask for a child's input when trying to make a system or routine easier to follow.
- Give your child one direction to follow at a time and gradually work up to two.
- Maintain a sense of humor.

## In Conclusion

Sometimes the most challenging things we endure in life are also the ones that teach us the most. This can be true of raising and living with an ADHD child. As a whole, the process of helping such a child turn his difficulties into assets can be highly enriching. Every step forward can seem a milestone. Parents and siblings can change and grow, learning patience, stress management, and how to turn frustration into positive action. Lastly, receiving a child's appreciation of a parent's understanding and caring can be the most rewarding experience of all.

# Index

# Suggested Reading

Hartman, Thom. *Attention Deficit Disorder: A Different Perception* (Lancaster, PA: Underwood-Miller Books, 1993).

Feingold, Ben. *Why Your Child Is Hyperactive* (New York: Random House, 1975).

Briggs, Dorothy. *Your Child's Self-Esteem* (New York: Doubleday, 1975).

Clarke, Jean. *Self-Esteem: A Family Affair* (New York: Harper & Row, 1978).

# Resources

*Feingold Association of the United States*, 127 East Main Street, Ste. 106, Riverhead, NY 11901 • 800-321-3287. Call or write for information on the Feingold program.

*Sensory Integration International (The Ayres Clinic)*, 1602 Cabrillo Avenue, Torrance, CA 90501 • 310-320-9986. Call or write for information on sensory defensiveness.

*International Health Foundation*, P.O. Box 3494, Jackson, TN 38303 • 901-427-8100. Call or write for information on nutrition and allergies.

# About the Author

Diana Hunter is an author, speaker, and consultant on the subjects of hyperactivity and attention deficits. Her background includes over twelve years of related research and studies. A hyperactive adult and parent of two hyperactive children, she is experienced in using drug-free approaches to manage hyperactivity and inattention both in self-management and parenting.

Ms. Hunter resides in Ft. Lauderdale, Florida.

# Order Form

Copies of *The Ritalin-Free Child* are only $12.95, plus $3.00 shipping and handling. Florida residents add 6% sales tax.

Name_____

Address_____

City_____State_____Zip_____

     ____ copies @ $12.95 =       _____

     6% Sales Tax (FL res. only)   _____

     Shipping/Handling

     ($3.00 first copy,

     $2.00 each add'l copy)     _____

     TOTAL        _____

**Mail your order to:**

**CONSUMER PRESS, INC.**
Order Department RFC
13326 Southwest 28th Street
Ft. Lauderdale, FL 33330-1102

**For credit card orders call:** 800-266-5752

*Visit Our Website at*
**http://members.aol.com/BookGuest**
*or E-mail us at*
**BookGuest@aol.com**

☐  Please add my name to your mailing list for upcoming titles.